SAS FORCES

EXTREME FITNESS

SAS AND SPECIAL FORCES

EXTREME FITNESS

MILITARY WORKOUTS AND FITNESS CHALLENGES
FOR MAXIMISING PERFORMANCE

CHRIS McNAB

amber
BOOKS

This paperback edition first published in 2023

First published in 2015

Published by
Amber Books Ltd
United House
London N7 9DP
United Kingdom
www.amberbooks.co.uk
Instagram: amberbooksltd
Pinterest: amberbooksltd
Twitter: @amberbooks

ISBN: 978-1-83886-296-1

Project Editor: Michael Spilling
Design: MRM Graphics
Picture Research: Terry Forshaw
Illustrations: Tony Randell

Printed in the USA

Picture Credits
All photographs courtesy U.S. Department of Defense.

CONTENTS

INTRODUCTION

I am a relative latecomer to the world of endurance events. Having invested much time in intense martial arts training and competition during my early–mid 20s, I then suffered the all-too-familiar drop in fitness during my late 20s and early 30s as the pressures of family and career crowded in. The stamina of my youth began to drain away slowly, but the desire to stay in shape nagged in the background.

The turnaround came in my mid 30s, when following some health

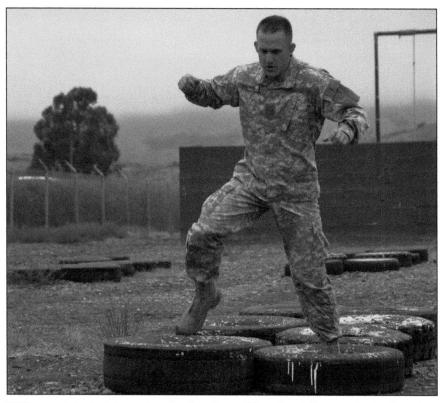

Military-style training aims to develop all levels of fitness, including the physical coordination required for this tyre-sprint obstacle.

problems I accepted that there were no excuses for a sluggish lifestyle. I decided to take up running in a serious way, and as I lived in Wales – one of the more undulating regions of the U.K. – this almost certainly meant I would become a hill runner.

I started small, with runs of less than 5km (3 miles), by pushing myself up the minor mountain just a mile from my front door. Playing the long game, I added small amounts of distance with each run, and started tackling new peaks. The biggest surprise was how much and how quickly I was hooked. I felt energized and renewed, and experienced the euphoria of conquering peaks and distances that just weeks before felt unobtainable. Soon I was running for hours not minutes, up slopes that bordered on climbs, tracking through the countryside of Wales. The new surge of fitness spurred me to add

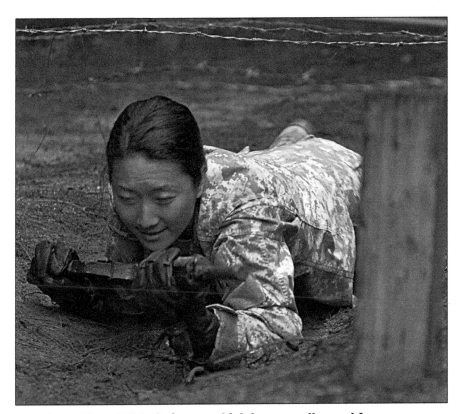

By using military PT techniques, which have an all-round focus on physical development, you will vastly increase fitness levels.

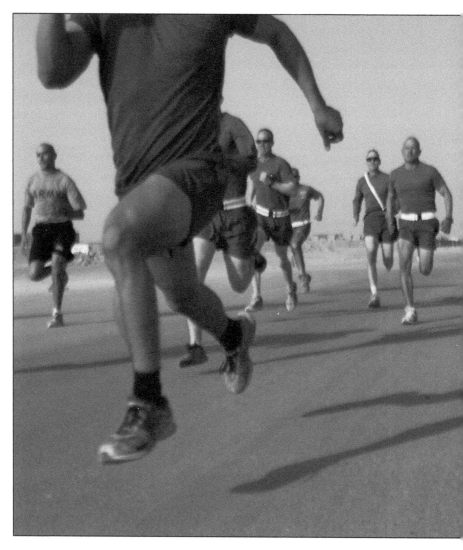

other activities, including weight training and circuit-training. By the time I reached 40, I was fitter than I had ever been in my life.

A particular inspiration for my activities was the military. As a military historian, as well as a sports enthusiast, I have always been slightly in awe of the incredible physical feats that soldiers perform, either in battle or in training. I run miles up mountains, but soldiers

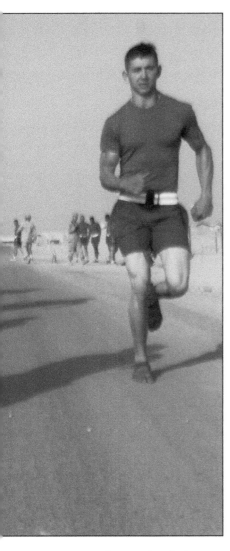

Military selection programmes demand superb aerobic endurance fitness, often fostered by long-distance runs.

testing every aspect of the soldier's physical and mental courage nearly to destruction. Furthermore, the military has over the years developed vast expertise in the art of bringing people to the peak of their physical condition. In effect, armies run the largest fitness programmes in the world, globally taking thousands of men and women to exceptional levels of performance every year. Because of these programmes, there are few better organizations to teach us about how to develop extreme fitness.

This book is about developing your physical condition to its limits in sports ranging from running through to rowing. The advice is both practical (based on the latest research and expert advice) and mental – those who possess extreme fitness need as much mental grit as bodily stamina. At every step of the way, we shall take on board lessons and insight from the military, particularly its Special Forces, whose personnel are exceptional endurance athletes. By adopting this perspective, the civilian athlete will discover new ways in which to excel, and tackle challenges that previously were beyond his or her reach.

do the same while carrying limb-deadening loads of pack and weaponry. In the world of the Special Forces, the training and selection regimes would in many cases halt a professional athlete, the trials

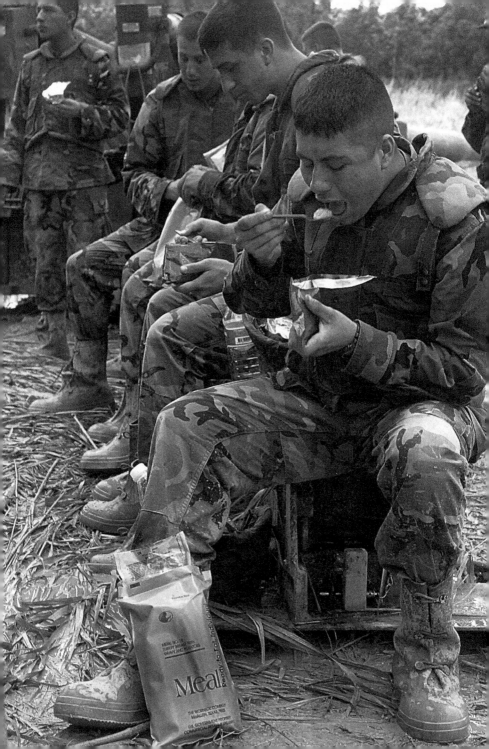

Developing extreme fitness is a laudable goal, but one that needs to be handled with some caution. There are no short-cuts to be taken here. There is no chemical, technology or technique that will take you from average fitness to super fitness in a matter of weeks. As we will see in this book, there are training programmes that can accelerate your physical development dramatically, but these will still require dedication and patience to implement for you to see the long-term rewards.

Before you embark on an extreme fitness programme, you need to do some basic physical housekeeping and some honest assessment. The fact is that high-impact training will place acute levels of stress upon your cardiovascular and muskuloskeletal systems. If you don't respect this fact by preparing your body through good lifestyle and fitness practices, the chances are that your training programme could end – and for good – in a nasty injury or other physical incident. Note that in basic military training, within every 100 male recruits an average of 6–12 will experience training injuries each month. In the Special Forces units, these rates can climb as high as 30 per 100. This data, provided

• •

Opposite: Adult diet should include all major food groups, as contained in these MRE packs.

1

Achieving the standards of physical fitness possessed by elite soldiers is not for the faint hearted. Before you launch into any high-impact training programme, you need to make an honest judgement about your capabilities.

Preparing the Body

Parkour Training

Parkour demands exceptional upper-body and core strength, as well as excellent spatial judgement. All techniques should be developed at safe heights before testing on elevated buildings.

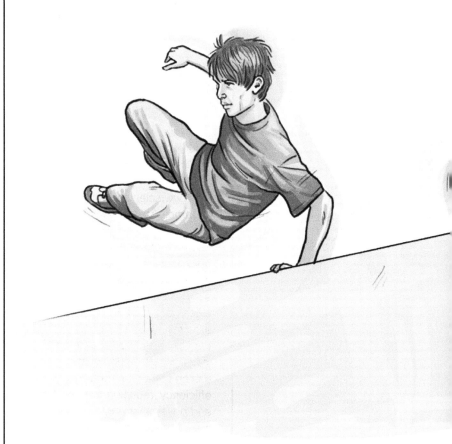

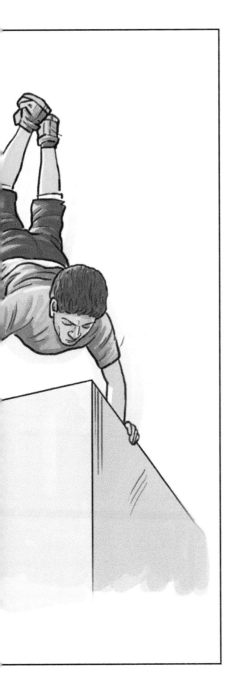

in the United States by researchers Kenton R. Kaufman, Stephanie Brodine and Richard Shaffer, also provided some firm conclusions about the core risk factors in why the rates of injury were so high:

> *Data collected show a wide variation in injury rates that are dependent largely on the following risk factors: low levels of current physical fitness, low levels of previous occupational and leisure time physical activity, previous injury history, high running mileage, high amount of weekly exercise, smoking, age and biomechanical factors. Kaufman, et al., 'Military Training-related Injuries'*

www.sciencedirect.com/science/article/pii/S0749379700001148

Much about this list is focused upon factors that take place outside the actual training regime. If, for example, the recruit has undertaken little exercise in civilian life before he enters the military world, the chances of injury during basic training increase significantly. Smoking also has an impact on cardiovascular efficiency, reducing both endurance and physical strength. Those who are carrying a previous injury run the risk of a repeat injury when the body is subjected to the new loads and strains of martial training.

Exhaustion

Pushing yourself too far, too fast, can have negative consequences on your fitness regime, including over-use injuries and exhaustion. Build up your training gradually, allowing for rest days and moderate exercise days in your training schedule at regular intervals.

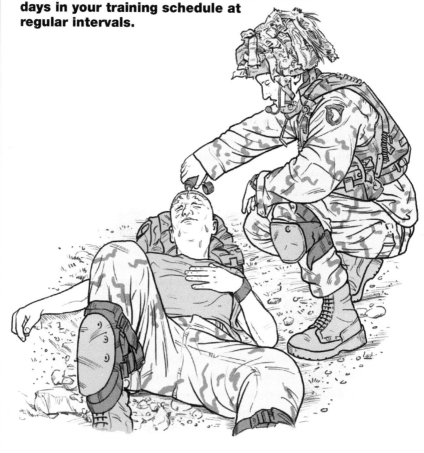

U.S. Armed Forces Tip – the Components of Physical Fitness

The components of physical fitness are as follows:

- Cardiorespiratory (CR) endurance – the efficiency with which the body delivers oxygen and nutrients needed for muscular activity and transports waste products from the cells.
- Muscular strength – the greatest amount of force a muscle or muscle group can exert in a single effort.
- Muscular endurance – the ability of a muscle or muscle group to perform repeated movements with a sub-maximal force for extended periods of time.
- Flexibility – the ability to move the joints (elbow or knee, for example) or any group of joints through an entire, normal range of motion.
- Body composition – the amount of body fat a soldier has in comparison to his total body mass.

– FM 21-20, *Physical Fitness Training, 1-3*

The moral of this information is that before you start extreme training, do an honest and thorough audit of your current health. This procedure is not to dissuade you from ambitious fitness goals, but to ensure that you tailor-design your programme to your physical needs.

Lifestyle

Lifestyle choices are absolutely critical to your fitness programme, as indiscipline in one area of your life can wipe out the benefits of discipline in another. Smoking is a habit you certainly need to cut out if you are to embark on military-style training. A study published in February 2001 in the United States assessed a total of 29,044 U.S. Air Force (USAF) personnel undergoing basic training over a 12-month period, and looked at the relationship between smoking and the rate of premature discharge from the service. The study found that 19.4 per cent of smokers were discharged, as against 11.8 per cent of non-smokers (Klesges et al.,

Effects of Smoking on Army Recruits

Studies of army recruits have yielded the following facts about smoking and training performance:

- Smokers were twice as likely to fail basic training as non-smokers.
- Smokers in endurance tests reach exhaustion earlier than non-smokers.
- Smokers ran a shorter distance in 12 minutes than non-smokers.
- Non-smokers ran an 80m (262ft) sprint in a significantly shorter time than smokers.
- Smokers in a 16km (10 mile) run were consistently slower than non-smokers.
- For every cigarette smoked per day, finishing time increased by 40 seconds.
- Smoking 20 a day increases the time to run 16km (10 miles) by 12 age years.

www.gasp.org.uk/articles-fitness-and-smoking-.htm

2001). The report's writers declared that 'the best single predictor of early discharge was smoking status', and that across the Department of Defense (DoD) smokers were costing the services more than $130 million.

Given the extent of public knowledge about the dangers of smoking, especially the dramatically increased risks of cancer, we do not need an elaborate argument for the reasons to stop. From the perspective of developing extreme fitness, cigarettes decrease cardiovascular efficiency – smokers have an increased heart rate and a reduced ability to take in and process oxygen, thus powers of endurance are weakened. Furthermore, the impact of smoking on muscular strength and flexibility means that smokers derive less benefit from exercise than non-smokers. Smoking also has a detrimental effect upon the health of bones, joints and tissue, resulting in extended injury recovery times when compared to non-smokers. Research

Muscle Groups

Your exercise regime should focus on developing all major muscle groups, to create a balanced physical strength.

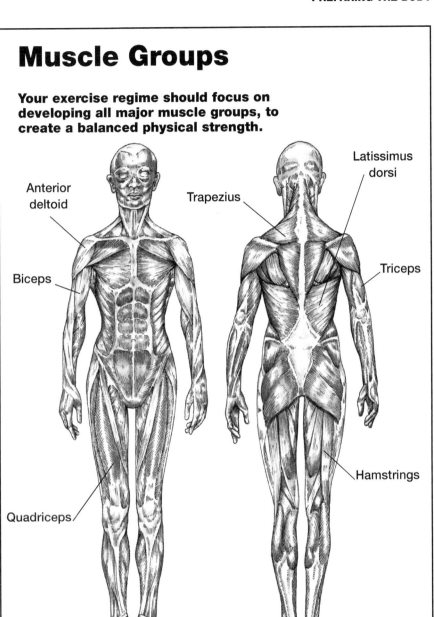

Anterior deltoid

Biceps

Quadriceps

Trapezius

Latissimus dorsi

Triceps

Hamstrings

Posture

Holding your body in the correct posture during exercise can prevent injury and increase the strength of core muscles. The vertical dotted lines in these pictures show the alignment of the spine weight being carried directly over the body's centre of gravity (the horizontal line). When standing, hold your body up straight and avoid tilting on either hip to prevent strain.

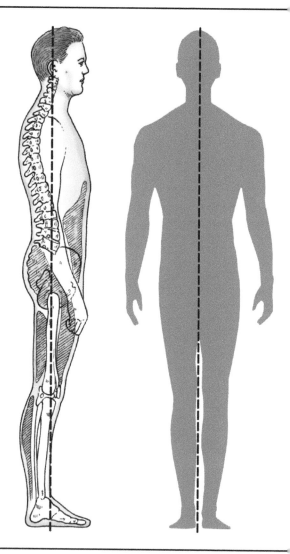

into people with tibia fractures, for example, found that the injuries of smokers took four additional weeks to heal when compared to those of non-smokers.

For these, and many other reasons, smoking has to stop before you attempt any extreme fitness programme. You must also look at your diet. Nutrition is the bedrock

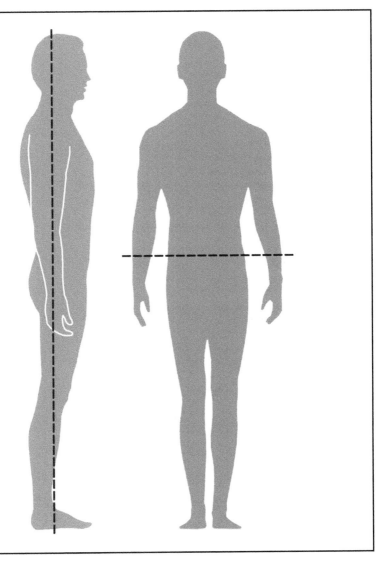

of any good fitness programme, as the food you eat provides not only the fuel for energy, but also has a central effect on the body's muscle development, fat-to-muscle ratio and your ability to combat certain diseases. Unfortunately, we are surrounded on a daily basis by large volumes of tempting but nutritionally empty foods. These foods, such

Effects of Smoking

Smoking not only hinders you from reaching your fitness goals, it can cause serious and potentially life-threatening diseases.

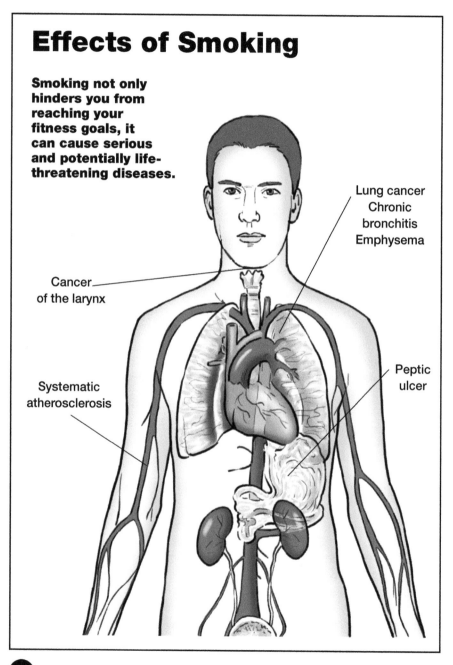

Lung cancer
Chronic
bronchitis
Emphysema

Cancer
of the larynx

Peptic
ulcer

Systematic
atherosclerosis

as low-cost burgers, take-outs, confectionary and carbonated drinks, are typically packed with sugar, salt and fat, and do little except satisfy a temporary craving. Long-term and excessive ingestion of these foods results in effects such as obesity, coronary heart disease, increased likelihood of some cancers, type 2 diabetes and general unfitness.

Understanding Calorie Intake

To understand the nature of the problem, and its solution, we have to understand the issue of calorie intake. A calorie is essentially a unit of energy produced by the digestion of food. We certainly need a base level of calorie intake just to maintain essential physiological processes – an adult male of average build requires about 2000–2500 calories a day, while a female needs around 1500–1800. If calorie intake exceeds calories consumed, then the result is typically weight gain. We can, however, increase the number of calories burned each day through exercise and activity. The equation for calculating the exact calorie consumption is complicated, and relates to areas such as body weight, metabolism and type of exercise, not just to the length of time spent performing the activity. As an illustration, however, the following figures are based on a 68kg (150lb) man performing the stated exercises over a 30-minute period:

- Aerobics
  (high impact)   238 cals
- Cycling (vigorous)   340
- Calisthenics (vigorous)   272
- Football (competitive)   306
- Martial arts   340
- Rock climbing   374
- Running (10km/h; 6mph)   340
- Skiing
  (cross-country, moderate)   272
- Swimming
  (freestyle, moderate)   238
- Walking (brisk)   129
- Weight training   109

As this list illustrates, the calories burnt according to the type of exercise vary considerably, from just over 100 to nearly 400. Yet regardless of the type of exercise, the calorific content of many foods can easily exceed even several hours of high-intensity exercise. For example, a large burger, chips and drink from a high-street fast-food chain can quite comfortably exceed 1300 calories; this calorie injection would take nearly four hours of running to burn off. A BLT baguette with butter, depending on size, is around 800 calories. A simple chocolate bar can add 500 calories in a couple of minutes.

From these quick figures, you can see instantly how easy it is for calorie intake to exceed calorie burn-off to a dramatic extent. This is evidenced by one of the great health crises of the modern age – obesity.

Calorie Requirements – Men

Knowing how many calories you should consume in a day enables you to control your intake. If you are increasing activity, you will need to increase calorie intake unless your immediate goal is to lose weight.

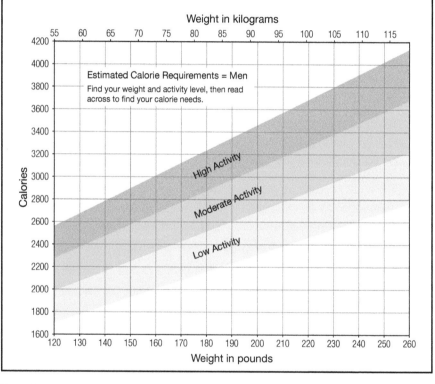

Data for 2009–2010 calculates that nearly 70 per cent of Americans are overweight, and the problem has now extended to the military. Over the last 15 years, the number of clinically obese soldiers serving in the U.S. Army has tripled. In the 10 months leading to December 2012, a total of 1625 soldiers were actually dismissed from the forces because of their obesity.

However, this unsettling picture is not always straightforward. Some soldiers point out that military

Obesity – United States

Obesity is defined by the World Health Organization as having a Body Mass Index (BMI) of 30 or more. The ideal BMI is between 18.5 and 24.9. Being obese puts you at greater risk of heart disease, stroke and type 2 diabetes. The table here shows U.S. obesity levels, 1960–2003.

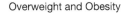

Overweight and Obesity

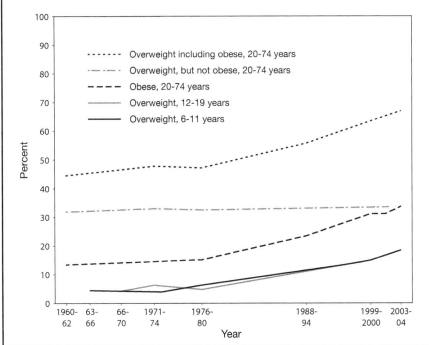

obesity often occurs following injuries suffered during extreme training sessions.

Nevertheless it does illustrate that even those individuals who are surrounded and immersed in a culture of physical fitness can still fall prey to obesity in such a calorie-rich environment.

Diet Management
During an intense diet/weight loss regime, especially one that the body has not experienced before, weight

loss can be quite rapid. The problem is that such regimes are typically not sustainable over a long period of time. For a start, any weight-loss programme that requires an unusual diet, particularly relying on proprietary supplements such as diet shakes, tends to become cloying and unsustainable over time. These restrictive diets frequently build up cravings for sweet, fattening foods, creating a mental pressure-cooker effect that results in excessive, rapid calorie consumption when the subject

A Square Meal

The importance of a healthy, well-balanced diet can not be underestimated when in training. In military circles, it also provides the opportunity for mental relaxation and camaraderie.

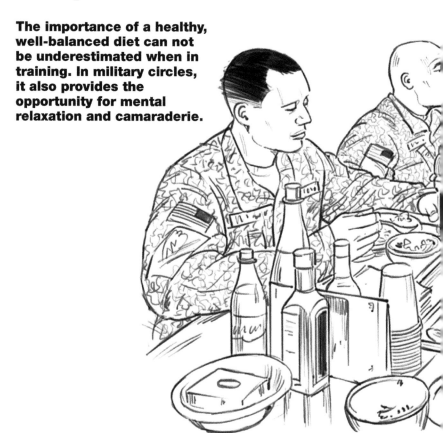

finally falls from the programme. But compounding this problem is an interesting dietary slingshot effect, revealed by recent research from the U.S. National Institutes for Health.

The research took to task the long-standing myth that if we cut our calorie consumption to 500 calories below our recommended allowance, then we can expect to lose 0.45kg (1lb) a week, or a total of 26kg (52lb) in a year. The U.S. researchers, using more accurate long-term modelling of how the human body behaves,

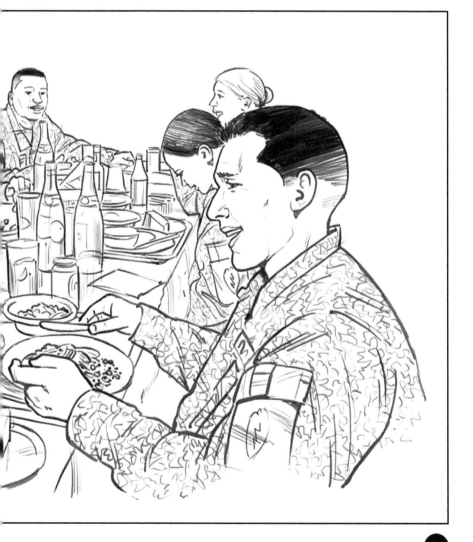

Weight-Loss Strategies

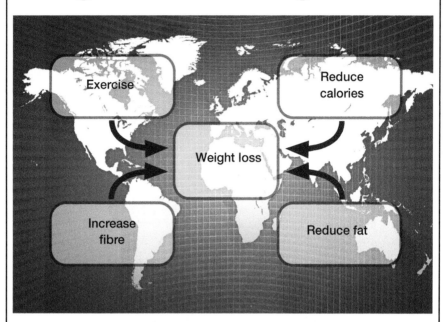

This diagram illustrates the fundamental principles of effective and consistent weight loss. Include all four elements of weight loss and excess weight will fall off.

found that weight loss takes place over a much longer duration than previously believed. In fact, the excess 26kg (52lb) would take an average of three years to shift with a 500-calorie reduction, allowing for metabolic changes as the subject's body adjusts to the progressive weight loss.

In reality, most people on strict diets see the maximum results after six months, but then 50–80 per cent of people subsequently not only put the weight back on, but also end up fatter than they were originally. The cause of this effect is that for an overlap period, the body continues to lose weight (because weight loss is a slow process) while the subject reverts to old dietary habits. This situation fools the subject into thinking that he will continue to lose weight even though he is eating heavily. Unfortunately, time will correct that misunderstanding – eventually the weight will go back on, and quickly.

Moderation and Habit

The point of the research above is not to discourage people from embarking on diets. Reducing calories and increasing exercise will indeed burn off excess weight, and the greater the effort the greater the weight loss. The key point however is sustainability. A well-balanced diet with calorie control should be a long-term habit, and not a short-term policy. To accomplish this, we need a simple approach to weight control that is both mentally and physically achievable, and which can become part of the general background to our lives for years, not just months.

Thankfully, this process is neither complicated nor onerous. The balance of all the sensible and properly researched dietary boils down to a few essential points. The first is that timeless piece of advice: 'Everything in moderation.' Contrary to what we might expect, a large, fatty burger is not in itself bad for our bodies. Rather, it is the excessive and frequent consumption of such foods that results in adverse health effects. In reality, if we eat a truly balanced diet, high in fruit, vegetables and lean protein, and consume high-fat, high-calorie foods infrequently, then our bodies will get everything they need. Simple calorie counting will inform

you of whether you are exceeding your daily limit; the internet and smartphone apps offer many different calorie-counting software options. One key point – make sure that you count absolutely everything you eat, including all those little 'snacks' that can add up to several hundred calories a day. Many a person has been perplexed by their inability to lose weight, not realizing that the culprit lies in the numerous minor meals and snacks eaten throughout the day.

Your aim is to make this diet of moderation and balance part of your ingrained daily habit. There are several ways in which you can use your imagination in this goal. First, adopt 'mindfulness' when it comes to food. This simply means that you are aware of every act of eating, rather than just blindly snacking when the urge takes hold. Whenever you are confronted by the need to eat, or tempted by a certain food, make yourself conscious of the moment and ask yourself questions such as:

Am I really hungry? If you ate a meal a short while ago, chances are you are simply tempted rather than hungry. Be particularly careful if you are feeling bored or stressed, as food might be a convenient route to alleviate these symptoms. You might also be misinterpreting thirst – have a good drink of water and you will often

Calorie Burning

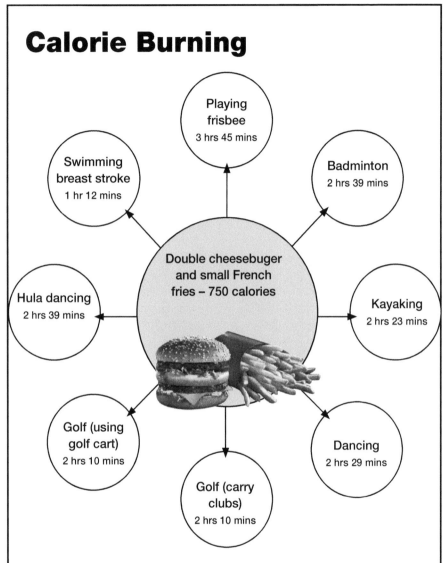

Playing frisbee
3 hrs 45 mins

Swimming breast stroke
1 hr 12 mins

Badminton
2 hrs 39 mins

Double cheesebuger and small French fries – 750 calories

Hula dancing
2 hrs 39 mins

Kayaking
2 hrs 23 mins

Golf (using golf cart)
2 hrs 10 mins

Golf (carry clubs)
2 hrs 10 mins

Dancing
2 hrs 29 mins

Be aware that the calorific value of many foods is extremely high, especially processed foods high in fat. The diagram above shows how long it takes to burn off a cheeseburger and French fries via various activities.

Eating at the Table

Eating at the table or with others means that you eat more slowly, which gives your body more time to register when you have had enough.

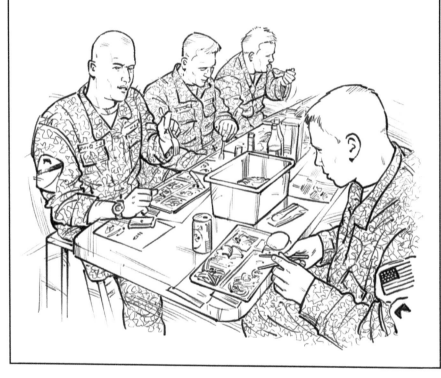

find your hunger abates. You can also try going for a walk – the movement shakes off some of that boredom and stress, and makes you less likely to turn to the food cupboard.

How much do I need to eat? Here we are in the realm of portion control, and it's a critical issue in the modern world. Nutritionists have noted that portion sizes and its calorific content has been inexorably creeping up in developed countries. Around 20 years ago, a two-slice portion of pizza amounted to about 500 calories; today it is closer to 850. Soda used to be sold only in 350ml (12oz) cans; now 500ml (17.5oz) bottles are more common, taking the calories from 145 to 242. Eating out has become a matter of epic indulgence. In many restaurants a meal consisting of a starter, main course and desert will easily total more than 2000 calories.

As a general rule, look to decrease your portion sizes, or at least substitute the high-fat foods with something less calorific (see feature box below for more tips).

How is the food prepared? Even a healthy food can be made into belt-busting stodge by its cooking method (think about the difference between a roasted chicken leg and one coated in breadcrumbs and deep-fried).

When choosing foods in a restaurant, follow the U.S. Department of Agriculture advice: 'Order steamed, grilled or broiled dishes instead of those that are fried or sautéed. Avoid choosing foods with the following words: creamy, breaded, battered or buttered.' Be careful with salad dressings – they

Tips for Reducing Your Portion and Calorie Consumption

- Prepare your food on a smaller plate. This simple psychological trick fools your mind into thinking that it is receiving more food than it actually is.
- Eat slowly, and be aware of the taste of every mouthful. Doing this will more quickly produce feelings of satiation.
- Shortly before eating a major meal, snack on something healthy, like a stick of celery or a low-fat yoghurt. This will take the edge off your hunger and help limit you indulging at the table.
- Think carefully about how food is prepared and cooked. Opt to fill your plate with foods that have been prepared healthily, such as boiling or grilling.
- When eating out, avoid oversized portions and choose foods that are prepared in a healthy way. Watch your drink consumption – unlimited refills of soda can add many hundreds of calories to your meal.
- At a restaurant, don't keep eating when you are full – ask for the remaining food to be packaged up in a take-out box.

Harmful Substances

Drugs and alcohol can have a damaging
effect on weight loss. Not only do you eat
more when intoxicated, most alcohol has a
high sugar and calorie content.
   Avoid all illegal drugs and moderate your
intake of alcohol to around one or two units
a day.

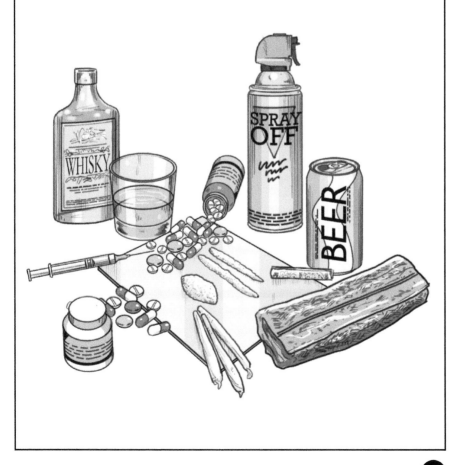

can transform a healthy salad into a fattening meal.

One helpful psychological tip to help you ensure good food habits is to imagine that a nutrition-wise sentry polices your mouth every time you go to eat. He asks all the right questions before he lets the food in. Try this technique for a 28-day period; research has shown that if you can follow a pattern of behaviour solidly for 28 days, there is a good chance that it will remain as a long-term habit.

Essential Foods

So what foods should you be eating to support your extreme fitness development? Fitness manuals are replete with advice about specialist diets, but as this book is for the general reader, and not necessarily the professional athlete, I again opt for a simple approach that is easier to sustain over time. The critical point is that you need to construct a diet from across the food groups to ensure that your body receives all the essential elements it needs for energy, a strong immune system and tissue repair. Everyone should aim to eat the correct balance of carbohydrates, proteins and fats.

Carbohydrates

Carbohydrates are used by your body to make glucose, which provides your muscles and body functions with energy. In this role, carbohydrates are obviously vital for those engaged in an intense fitness programme. You can find carbohydrates in fruit, vegetables, breads, cereals, grains, milk (and milk-based products) and anything sugary (cakes, sugar-rich drinks and confectionary). The problem is that not all carbohydrates have the same nutritional value.

Simple carbohydrates have a chemical structure consisting of one or two sugars, and they include the sugars in many fruits plus the refined sugars used in the production of sweets, cakes, jam, biscuits, etc. These sugars are broken down very quickly by the body to provide an immediate jolt of energy, so they do have a practical use for providing an extra boost when stamina flags. The problem is that this energy doesn't last for long, and foods heavy in refined sugars provide few other benefits for the body.

Complex carbohydrates, by contrast, have three of more sugars linked structurally in a chain, and take longer for the body to digest. The result is that complex carbohydrates release their energy over a long period, something useful for endurance events. Many complex carbohydrates also provide high levels of fibre, which helps to establish an efficient digestion system. You can find complex

Working Out

A combination of strength- and stamina-building exercises will result in the most useful workout. This dumbell exercise strengthens the lats and abdominal muscles.

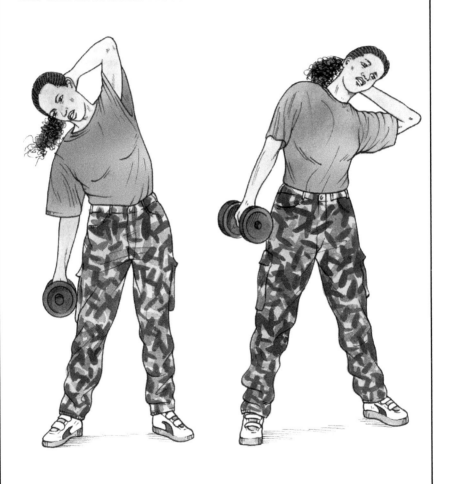

carbohydrates in foods such as vegetables, wholemeal bread, wholegrain cereals, oatmeal, grains, brown rice and pasta, beans and lentils. Given their benefits, plus their increased contribution of vitamins and minerals (see below), complex carbohydrates should form the bulk of your carbohydrate consumption, with simple carbohydrates used only as a temporary energy pick-up. The United States Air Force Dietetics (USAFD) organization recommends that 45–65 per cent of your total calorific intake is in the form of carbohydrates, with at least half your grain intake in the form of whole grains.

Proteins

Proteins are, like carbohydrates, another essential component of your diet. Proteins, made up of amino acids, are the structural building blocks of our bodies right down to the cellular level. These proteins are constantly broken down and replaced, and dietary protein intake is therefore critical not only to fundamental body functions, but also recovery from fitness activities and improvements in muscle strength. Protein is found in the following foods: meat (including poultry and fish), legumes, eggs, tofu, nuts and seeds, milk/milk products and (in small amounts) grains and some types of fruit and vegetables.

In athletes, protein demands are high, and the USAFD recommendation is that protein constitutes 10–35 per cent of your diet. Athletes – and especially weight lifters and bodybuilders – often use protein supplements in order to help the rapid development of muscle mass. Typically these come in the form of pills or a powdered formula for adding to drinks. Whey-based proteins appear to be the superior form of supplement (although they are not well-suited to people who are lactose intolerant).

I treat the subject of supplements with some caution. Protein supplements do indeed seem to aid muscle development and recovery with few side effects, at least in the short and medium term. A controlled scientific trial in 2003 tested protein supplements on U.S. Marines undergoing rigorous training at the U.S. Marine Corps Base, Parris Island. The protein-supplemented group (as opposed to placebo and control groups) appeared to experience clear benefits:

[They] had an average of 33 per cent fewer total medical visits, 28 per cent fewer visits due to bacterial/viral infections, 37 per cent fewer visits due to muscle/joint problems and 83 per cent fewer visits due to heat exhaustion... Muscle soreness immediately post-exercise was reduced by protein

Food Types

This diagram shows the variety of food groups you should eat every day for optimal health. By varying the types of foods within each group, your intake of carbohydrates, proteins, vitamins and minerals will support your training regime.

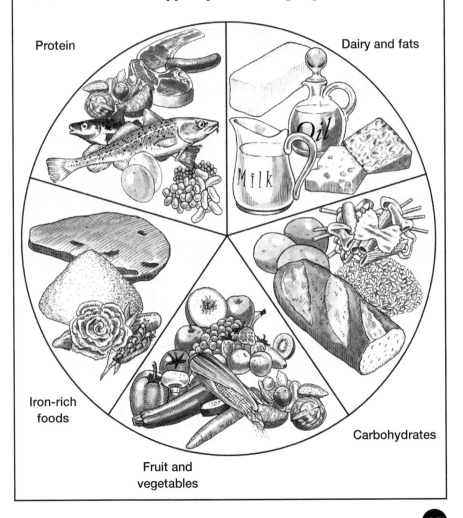

Protein

Dairy and fats

Iron-rich foods

Carbohydrates

Fruit and vegetables

Sources of Fats

Fats are an essential part of any diet. Unsaturated fats, such as those found in fish and nuts, can help lower cholesterol and prevent heart disease. Saturated fats found in butter and oil are high in calories and have few health benefits, thus should be limited in your overall diet.

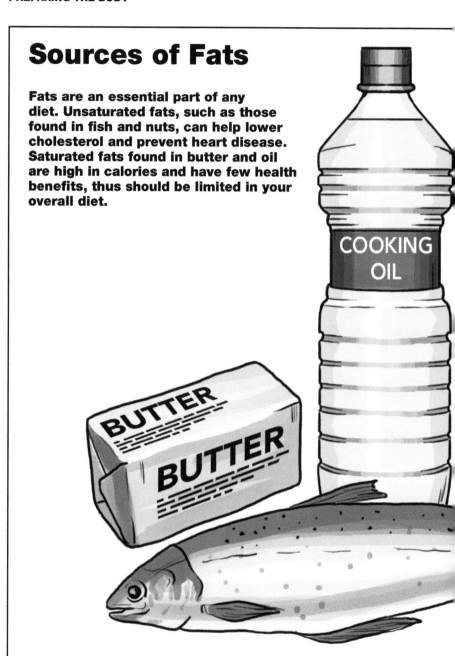

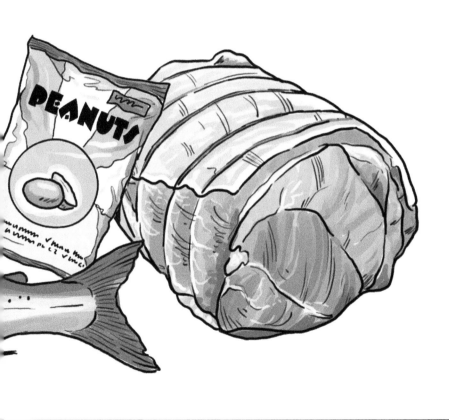

The Press-up

An effective press-up
should feature a full range
of motion, the arms being
at 90 degrees at the lowest
part of the movement.
Keep the body straight and
aligned at all times during
the movement.

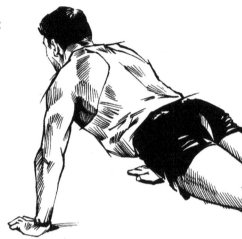

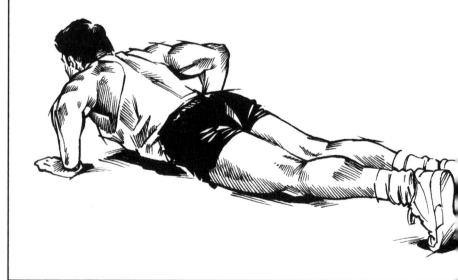

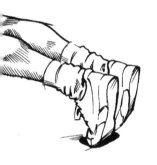

supplementation vs. placebo and control groups on both days 34 and 54. Post-exercise protein supplementation may not only enhance muscle protein deposition but it also has significant potential to positively impact health, muscle soreness and tissue hydration during prolonged intense exercise training, suggesting a potential therapeutic approach for the prevention of health problems in severely stressed exercising populations.

– www.ncbi.nlm.nih.gov/
pubmed/14657039

On this basis, protein supplements have a clear role in post-exercise recovery. Treat any supplement with caution, however. Many are recent additions to dietary control, and the long-term effects are yet to be seen. As with the dietary advice above, use them in moderation and place your confidence more in a well-rounded conventional diet. Only purchase supplements from approved dealers, and check out several reviews of the product (including any independent medical articles) before using it. It is also a good idea to consult a doctor before embarking on a supplement programme – one that produces beneficial results for one person could cause medical harm in another.

Fats

Beyond proteins we move into the realm of fats. Fats are traditionally regarded as the bogeyman of the dietary world on account of their primary responsibility for the obesity epidemic plaguing modern society. The problem is that fats both taste good and are a highly concentrated source of calories. They also come in different varieties with contrasting properties. On the 'bad fats' side are saturated fats and trans fats. Foods high in saturated fats include fatty meat, processed meat products (such as pies and sausages), butter, cheese, cream and much confectionary, biscuits and cakes. Consuming these products heavily and repeatedly can result in the build up of cholesterol in the blood, a major factor in the cause of heart disease and stroke in later life.

Trans fats occur in small quantities in meat and dairy products, and in higher levels in foods containing hydrogenated vegetable oils. They are similarly bad for raising cholesterol levels, although better food production standards means that the levels present in our food tend to be very low.

On the credit side of fats are the unsaturated varieties. They are found in in sunflower and olive oils, nuts, seeds and in oily fish (such as salmon, mackerel and sardines). Unsaturated fats can actually lower blood cholesterol levels, which is one reason why Mediterranean diets tend to be far healthier than those in northern Europe. The Omega-3 essential fatty acids found in oily fish, and Omega-3-enhanced products, can deliver even more benefits. A U.S. Army Food Service presentation on the positive effects of Omega-3 include:

- *Reduce risk of heart disease*
- *Lower blood pressure*
- *Reduce risk of depression, bipolar disorder, ADHD*
- *Possible protective role in Traumatic Brain Injury (TBI) and Post Traumatic Stress Disorder (PTSD)*

www.quartermaster.army.mil/jccoe/operations_directorate/cspd/Workshop_Information/Nutrition_Brief.pdf

Although fats can cause serious health problems, they remain necessary for optimal health and are important for athletic endurance. Fats are an important source of energy for extended aerobic activities. As we have seen, your fat intake should be heavily weighted towards unsaturated fats, with less then 10 per cent of calories from saturated fats. Also, try to replace solid fats with oils (olive and sunflower) where possible.

Vitamins and Minerals

In addition to the sustenance from

Energy Products

Energy products such as bars, gels or drinks can provide useful, concentrated boosts of energy when you most need them.

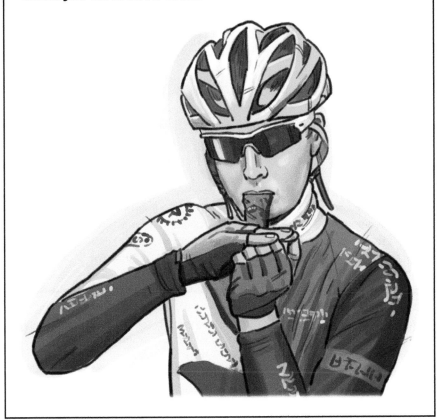

carbohydrates, proteins and fats, the human body also requires a broad spectrum of vitamins and minerals to function at optimal levels. Each of these vitamins and minerals makes its own contribution to health.

Vitamin D, for example (conveniently obtained from exposure to sunlight as well as from diet), promotes calcium absorption, ensuring that we have good bone strength and development. (The disease rickets, resulting in bone deformations, occurs from Vitamin D deficiency.) Vitamin C, obtained from citrus fruits, peppers, broccoli, potatoes and many other sources, keeps cells healthy and maintains connective tissue. Good iron sources include meat, cereals, beans, lentils and spinach. The functions of iron in the human body include efficient oxygen transportation in the blood and the regulation of cell growth and differentiation, and those without adequate iron (a condition known as iron deficiency anaemia) experience symptoms such as fatigue, dizziness, weakness, mood changes and poor immune function.

Simply having a balanced diet will ensure that you are getting all of your essential vitamins and minerals. Taking a daily supplement will also cover all the necessary bases, although never rely on a supplement as a substitute for a good diet – good food provides you with an array of benefits, more than a simple tablet can deliver.

In-training Nutrition

The discussion above has focused on how to establish good dietary habits to support your general health and fitness. These principles remain the bedrock of the nutrition advice for this book, as good general health is the primary support for developing fitness at all levels. Yet this book is about extreme fitness, and there is no doubt that engaging in punishing endurance activities may result in the need to warp and adapt normal dietary principles. The fact is that your calorie intake will likely have to increase significantly to cope with the extra demands on your body. During U.S. Navy SEAL training, recruits can be consuming some 7000 calories a day – more than three times the recommended limit – and still lose weight. (Admittedly such situations are rare, or of short duration.)

If you find that your training regime is producing dramatic weight loss, then you might simply need to increase the amount of calories you eat to compensate. Don't do this with junk food, however, but focus on high-quality carbohydrates and proteins. Several weeks before a big event, begin the process of 'carb loading' – building up your carbohydrate reserves to draw on during the challenge ahead. Do this by consuming carbohydrates with a low glycemic index (GI), meaning that they are absorbed by the body more slowly than high-GI carbs. Wholegrain rice and pasta and porridge are good options, supplemented by lean meats and plenty of fresh fruit and vegetables.

On the day of an actual event you naturally want to avoid overburdening your digestive system with a hefty meal just prior to the challenge. Instead, take in some

Unusual Leisure Exercises

Exercise does not have to be boring. You are much more likely to stick to your training and feel the benefits if you enjoy it. Activities such as hip-hop dancing (shown here) skateboarding, parkour and surf flying are growing in popularity.

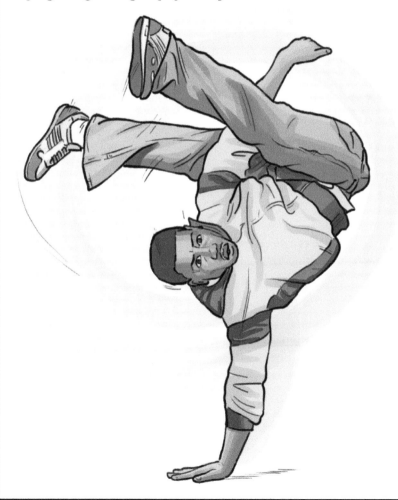

Lying Quad Stretch

The lying quad stretch utilizes a towel to stretch the front of the thigh. Extend the stretch to its maximum extent, then hold in place for 10 seconds, relaxing the muscle as you do so. Repeat on the other side.

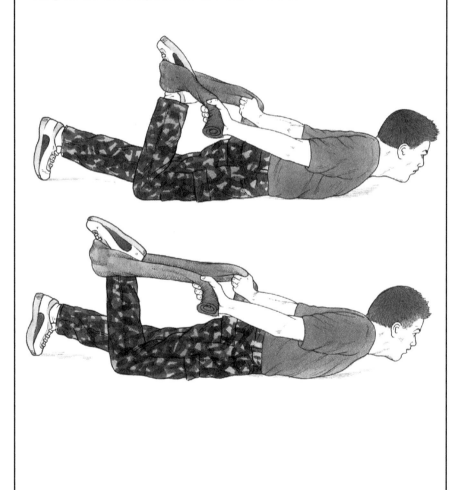

good low-GI snacks, such as a chicken sandwich on wholemeal bread, peanut butter sandwiches, fruit or porridge, a few hours before the race. During the event itself, if it takes place over many hours you are also going to need to replenish your energy reserves as you run out of carb energy. Here high-GI foods such as confectionary, fruit (particularly bananas and oranges) – dried or fresh – honey and energy bars are best, as these will deliver a rapid and much-needed shock of energy. Aim to take on board about 140 calories of carbs for every hour of exertion. You can also utilize high-carb sports gels, which provide an energy source in a more convenient package than many foods. Note that these typically have to be ingested with water, so ensure that you have access to plenty of fluids. A single gel can be taken about every 30–45 minutes during the endurance challenge.

Controlling your diet ensures that you maximize your body's energy reserves and also that you don't undo all your good work exercising through inappropriate eating. The chapters that follow will make further comments about nutrition in relation to individual extreme fitness activities. Here, however, we will make some more observations about ways in which you can prepare yourself for intense or prolonged fitness challenges.

Flexibility

The topic of flexibility is one that has been complicated by recent research. In the past it was believed that all athletes should invest in pre-event stretching both as a way to prevent injury and to improve performance. While there are definite physical benefits to stretching, research has thrown up some unsettling results, particularly in relation to running.

For example, some studies have shown that stretching before endurance runs actually seems to *increase* the likelihood of injury, possibly through overextension of joints (a similar effect has been seen in American football players, who develop excessive hamstring flexibility that in turn can create knee instability). In contrast, professional football players who develop good groin and hip flexibility do seem to be more protected from injuries to these areas.

Although much work remains to be done, some important conclusions do seem to be emerging. The first is that static stretching, or the type frequently performed prior to fitness challenges, actually seems to do little in terms of injury prevention or performance improvements, unless your specific sport requires excellent flexibility, such as martial arts. Instead, what is critical is that the athlete has a good range of mobility across

Stretching Tips

- Gently pull out of a stretch if you feel any burning or tearing sensations in the muscle.
- Don't 'bounce' a stretch further than you can comfortably handle. There is a role for what is known as 'ballistic stretching' (using momentum to stretch a muscle), but it should only be performed once the muscles are thoroughly warmed up, and it should not be pushed so hard that it produces sudden injury.
- When performing partner-assisted stretches, implement a series of short, clear instructions so that your partner does not push you beyond your physical limits.
- Warm up gently before stretching. Jogging on the spot gently or performing some light aerobic exercises, such as star jumps, will raise the temperature of your muscles and make them more pliant during the stretching process.

the full range of limb movement required specifically for a particular sport. In the following chapters we will highlight stretches that can be performed between training sessions to improve active range-of-movement (ROM), but the box feature above provides some general rules you should apply to all your stretching efforts.

Equipment

Every sport has it's own set of specialized equipment. For many sportsmen and women, acquiring and using this equipment is part of the fun and challenge of the sport itself.

In extreme fitness sports it is crucial that you have the right equipment, and the very best that you can afford. When buying any new item, do your research thoroughly, not only looking at product reviews but also internet forums, where you will often find first-hand accounts of how the product performed under actual event conditions. If you are unsure about what to purchase, buy your products from good sports shops with expert staff (you may have to travel some distance to find these).

If any of your equipment is mechanical (such as a bicycle or rowing machine, for example), also

Hamstring Stretch

While performing the hamstring stretch, keep looking forward to avoid hunching your back and putting strain on your lower spine. Breathe out every time you increase the stretch.

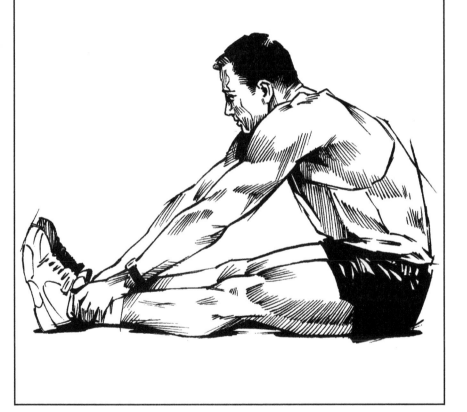

ensure that it is properly maintained. The components of any fitness machine will have a finite life, and if you are into extreme events then the equipment might need professional maintenance every few months. In particular, be careful to check for wear and tear around moving parts such as belts, cables and bearings afterward.

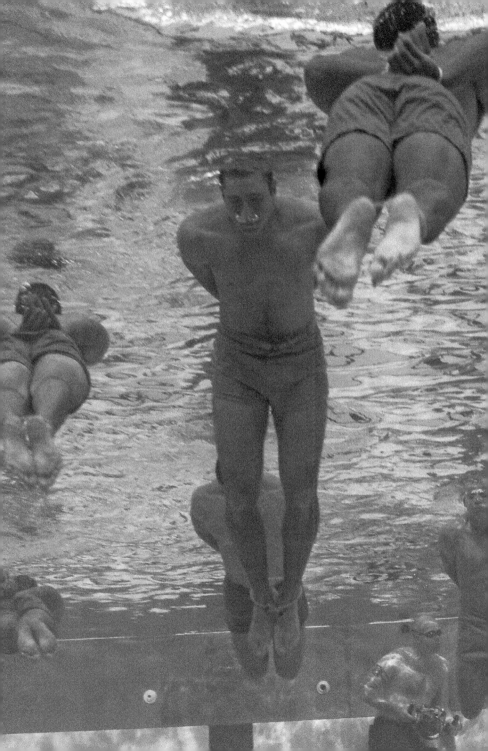

2

Military Workouts

There is much bravado among military enthusiasts, and among the military community itself, about which Special Forces units have the toughest physical training regimes. In truth, the selection and training programmes for all elite units tend to be gruelling in the extreme, hence the elevated failure rates for those attempting to join. In the U.S. Marine Corps, about 40 per cent of those who enlist fail the recruitment process. For U.S. Army Special Forces, failure rates hover at around 60–70 per cent, while for units such as the Special Air Service (SAS), British Royal Marines and U.S. Navy SEALs, failure rates are at an unforgiving 75–90 per cent. (All these figures vary, of course, according to the class going through the recruitment process.)

Not all of those who fail to make the grade do so by flunking the physical tests. Some simply don't pass the initial medical (often much to their surprise), while others have insurmountable problems adjusting to the discipline required. Yet a lion's share doesn't make the grade because they can't achieve the physical challenges within the training programme. Those who turn up for Special Forces selection without high levels of all-round fitness are doomed to failure. Physical Training Instructors

• •

Opposite: Drown-proofing is one of the many parts of SEAL stress training that new recruits undergo.

U.S. Army Physical Fitness Manual – Principles of Exercise

Regularity. To achieve a training effect ... one should strive to exercise ... at least three times a week. Infrequent exercise can do more harm than good. Regularity is also important in resting, sleeping and following a good diet.

Progression. The intensity (how hard) and/or duration (how long) of exercise must gradually increase to improve the level of fitness.

Balance. To be effective, a program should include activities that address all the fitness components, since overemphasizing any one of them may hurt the others.

Variety. Providing a variety of activities reduces boredom and increases motivation and progress.

Specificity. Training must be geared toward specific goals. For example, soldiers become better runners if their training emphasizes running. Although swimming is great exercise, it does not improve a two-mile-run time as much as a running program does.

Recovery. A hard day of training for a given component of fitness should be followed by an easier training day or rest day for that component and/or muscle group(s) to help permit recovery. Another way to allow recovery is to alternate the muscle groups exercised every other day, especially when training for strength and/or muscle endurance.

Overload. The workload of each exercise session must exceed the normal demands placed on the body in order to bring about a training effect.

– U.S. Army, *FM 21-20, 1–4*

(PTIs) emphasize to candidates that Special Forces training is not intended to take unfit people to super-fit levels, but relies on the candidates bringing a lot of strength, endurance and stamina to the table.

SEAL Training

A good benchmark for understanding Special Forces training, and the lessons it provides for developing extreme fitness, is the U.S. Navy SEALs Basic Underwater Demolition/ SEAL (BUD/S) programme. This infamous, punishing 24-week ordeal must be passed by those who wish to become SEALs, taking the candidates to the very limits of physical endurance in both land and aquatic environments.

Below: SEALS regularly train in tough field conditions to develop their endurance and stamina.

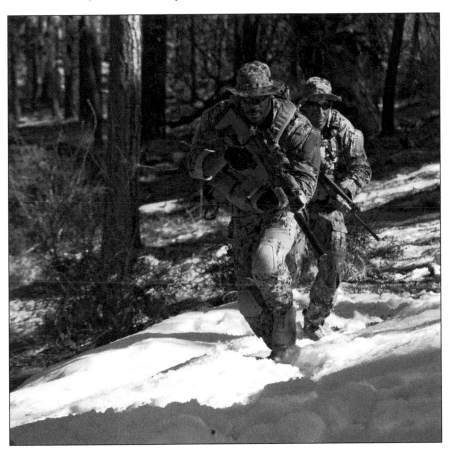

U.S. Navy SEALS
Deep Water Swimming

Swimming is an excellent aerobic exercise that uses many muscle groups. Deep water swimming is also great for building stamina and lung capacity.

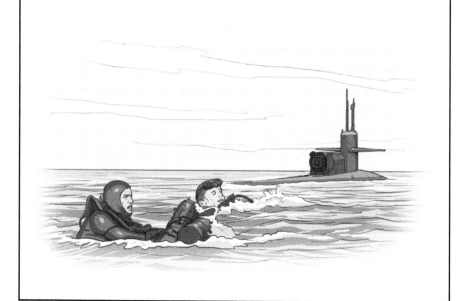

Not everyone can become a SEAL in the first place. Recruitment is restricted to U.S. males between 17 and 28 years of age (although there are waivers for candidates aged 29–30). All require uncorrected vision of at least 20/70 in the worst eye and 20/40 in the best. The candidates need to be educated to high-school level, and have to score the appropriate levels on the Armed Services Vocational Aptitude Battery (ASVAB), which is designed to test mental abilities in a range of cognitive fields. They also undergo a Computerized-Special Operations

Resilience Test (C-SORT), a form of psychometric test that explores the candidate's mental toughness and defines his basic character type.

At this pre-recruitment stage, the candidate also has to perform an initial Physical Screening Test (PST) to ensure that he has the physical requirements to at least begin SEALs training. The PST breaks down as follows, with minimum and optimum time requirements shown in the table:

Note the composition of this PST. By testing swimming, strength exercises and running, the PST delivers an all-round fitness evaluation. This is a key point about Special Forces fitness programmes to which we shall return frequently. An elite soldier needs to have a complete fitness profile – there can be no weak links in his physical armour. The SEALs clarify this point in their *Naval Special Warfare Physical Training*

Test	Minimum requirement	Optimum requirement
Swim 457m (1500ft/500yd)	12:30	9:00
Push-ups	50	90
Curl-ups a.k.a. sit-ups	50	85
Pull-ups	10	18
Run 2.4km (1.5 miles)	10:30	09:30

Swim 457m (1500ft/500yd) (timed breast stroke or side stroke) – rest 10 minutes
Push-ups (max set in two minutes) – two minute rest
Curl-ups a.k.a sit-ups (max set in two minutes) – two minute rest
Pull-ups (max set in two minutes) – ten minute rest
Run a distance of 2.4km (1.5 miles) (timed dressed in running shorts and shoes)

Guide, designed to help interested candidates improve their fitness in readiness for the PST and BUD/S:

Most of your cardiovascular exercise should focus on running and swimming, and your strength and calisthenics training should be done to develop the necessary muscular strength and endurance for maximum pull-ups, push-ups and sit-ups as they are necessary for success at BUD/S. Cross-training such as cycling, rowing and hiking is useful to rehabilitate an injury, to add variety or to supplement your basic training. Work to improve your weakest areas. If you are a solid runner but a weak swimmer, don't spend all your time running just because you are good at it. Move out of your comfort zone, and spend enough time in the water to become a solid swimmer as well. – NAVSOC, *Naval Special Warfare Physical Training Guide*, p.2

Types of Exercise

The advice here about 'move out of your comfort zone' is essential for anyone tackling extreme fitness challenges. It is often apparent how people can model their fitness on a limited range of exercises, then

Keeping Hydrated

A mere two per cent drop in body fluids can result in physical symptoms such as headaches, fatigue, dizziness and lowered blood pressure.

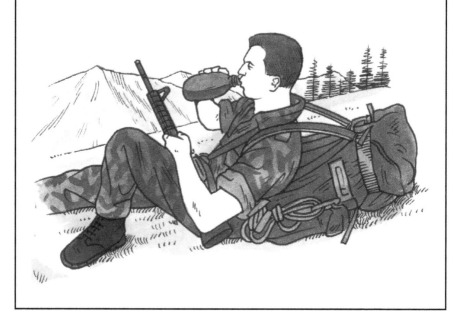

wonder why they feel so unfit when they try a new form of challenge. I, for example, might be able to run to the top of the most precipitous hills with vigour, but multiple lengths of a swimming pool using breaststroke seem to drain me, drawing as they do on a different range of muscle groups. For this reason, make sure you invest in what might be termed 'full-spectrum training', a physical regime that pushes into all the nooks and crannies of your physical development.

In basic terms, the four fundamental types of exercise you should pursue are: endurance, strength, balance and flexibility. Representative activities in these categories are as follows:

Type of exercise	Examples
Endurance	Running
	Swimming
	Biking
	Hiking
	Dancing
	Racquet sports
Strength	Weight training
	Resistance exercises (push-ups, pull-ups)
	Lifting activities (heavy gardening, building)
Balance	Yoga
	Martial arts
	Pilates
Flexibility	Yoga
	Pilates
	General stretching routines

Running with Full Kit

Special forces soldiers are expected to have the endurance and strength to carry a 35kg (80lb) pack while running long distances, often over rugged terrain. This is an excellent, intensive whole body workout.

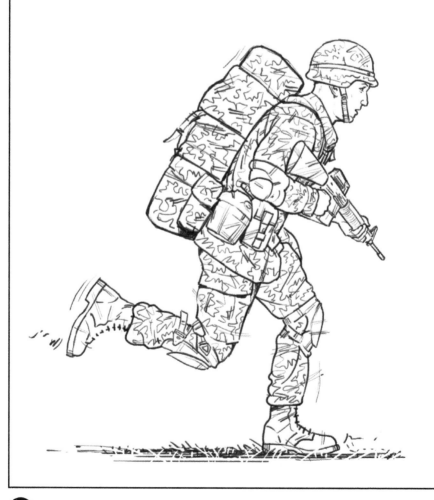

A good extreme fitness-training regime will typically utilize at least one activity from each category, or at least combined elements of different exercises into one routine. Within the endurance category, also think about mixing aerobic and anaerobic type activities. Aerobic activities are those that require oxygen to provide the fuel for muscles over prolonged periods. Running, swimming, cycling – indeed any activity in which you breath deeply and steadily over a prolonged period – is an aerobic activity. (One crude test for an aerobic activity is that while exercising you should be able to speak short sentences coherently.) However, some very high-intensity activities – sprinting or powerlifting, for example – require energy requirements beyond the capabilities of respiration. Under these circumstances, the muscles break down sugars to create energy. (This process in turn produces lactic acid, the chemical that results in limbs feeling heavy and fatigued at the end of a heavy session.)

Aerobic and Anerobic Training

Your exercise regime should include both aerobic and anerobic elements to produce a well-constructed fitness. Sometimes this can be achieved by two different types of exercise – mixing running and martial arts would be an example. However, you can also build aerobic and anerobic exercises into the same activity, by varying the intensity of effort. For example, if you mix regular 30-second sprints into an endurance run you create a form of interval training (raising your heart rate to near maximum for short periods of time between rest periods) that is excellent for both your stamina and for ancillary benefits such as weight loss.

The *Naval Special Warfare Physical Training Guide* gives some advice on the weekly training regime that potential SEAL candidates should pursue to develop their all-over body fitness. It summarizes a typical weekly workout as follows:

- *1 Long Slow Distance workout for both running and swimming*
- *1 Continuous High Intensity workout for both running and swimming*
- *1 Interval workout for both running and swimming*
- *4–5 Calisthenics Routines*
- *4–6 Strength Training Sessions – 2–3 each for upper and lower body*
- *4–5 Core Exercise Routines*
- *Daily Flexibility Routines*
- *Specific injury prevention exercises as needed*

    – NACSOC, *Naval Special Warfare Physical Training Guide*, p.2

This plan of action, while not even approaching the level of intensity that

Core Stability

The core muscles of the stomach, hips and mid to lower back are vital for increasing stability, flexibility, balance and quick reactions.

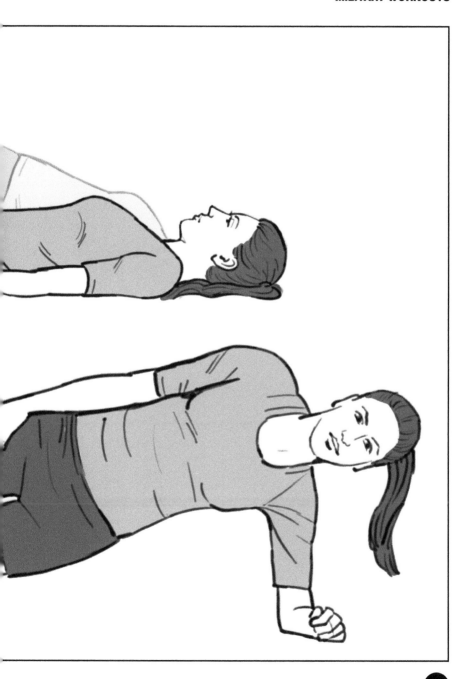

will face the recruits during BUD/S, still provides an excellent model for a weekly full-spectrum build-up. Mix any intense regime such as this with appropriate recovery time between activities. The 26-week programme daily programme recommended by the Naval Special Warfare Command (NSWC) features a cardio and a strength activity every day from Monday to Saturday, with Sunday being a day of complete rest and recovery. As Chapter 8 will insist, don't skimp on your recovery time, as this is the period in which your body strengthens and recuperates.

BUD/S

If a recruit ticks all pre-selection boxes satisfactorily, and also

U.S. Navy SEALs Tip – 'Bridge' Core Training Exercise

- Lie on back with knees bent and feet about 25cm (10in) from buttocks.
- Keep arms at sides or folded across the chest and keep the pelvis neutral.
- Raise the hips off the floor, creating a straight line between the knees, hips and shoulders.
- Lift the right foot off the floor and extend the leg until it is straight and creates a line from the shoulder through the hip, knee and foot.
- Meanwhile, support the body's weight by statically contracting the glutes and hamstring of the left leg. Make sure to keep the pelvis neutral and horizontal; don't let it dip toward the unsupported side.
- Hold the contraction for 3–4 seconds before lowering the pelvis to the floor with both feet near the buttocks in the original starting position.
- Lift the left foot off the floor and extend the leg while supporting the body's weight with the right leg in the same manner for 3–4 seconds. Continue to alternate between legs.

negotiates the security clearance requirements (including showing that they are of 'good moral character'), they can pass on to SEAL training proper. The first stage is the two-months of 'BUD/S Prep' held at the Naval Special Warfare Preparatory School in the Great Lakes, Illinois. The Preparatory School has various athletic facilities and it is intended to prepare the recruits for the ordeals of full BUD/S. At the outset, the PST outlined earlier is expanded to a higher level of intensity:

- 940m (3084ft) swim – with fins (20 minutes or under)
- Push-ups: at least 70 (two-minute time limit)
- Pull-ups: at least 10 (two-minute time limit)
- Curl-ups: at least 60 (two-minute time limit)
- 6.4km (4-mile) run – with shoes and pants (31 minutes or under)

Any recruit who fails these tests at this early stage is removed from the training programme and reassigned to other jobs within the U.S. Navy – there are few second chances in SEALs selection.

BUD/S Prep progressively raises the bar on the recruits' fitness levels, and is followed by a three-week 'Basic Orientation' phase at the Naval Special Warfare Center in Coronado, California. Again the pace of physical training accelerates, but this is only to accommodate the candidate for the real shock of BUD/S, which begins in earnest with the seven-week Basic Conditioning programme.

Basic Conditioning, despite its innocuous name, is the acid test of the individual's physical strength. Every day consists of ever-harder runs (with and without full kit), obstacle courses, swimming challenges (swimming pool and sea swims of many kilometres distance) and obstacle courses. Special tortures include crawls for hundreds of metres through thick, freezing coastal mud, or lying in the surf until the body temperature drops to near hypothermic levels.

Surviving 'Hell Week'

The fourth week of Basic Conditioning culminates in the body shock known as 'Hell Week'. In five-and-a half days, the candidates will sleep for a total of four hours, and exercise for an average of 20 hours per day. Candidates will also run some 320km (200 miles), and swim dozens of kilometres while exhausted and energy depleted. Such is the energy expenditure during this phase that despite consuming up to 7000 calories a day, each man will have lost weight by the end of Hell Week.

The dropout rate during Hell Week can reach 75 per cent of the candidates. PTIs will offer seductive promises of warm food and blankets to the exhausted recruits if they

Assault Course

Building elements
of competition into
training can give you
the extra incentive
sometimes needed to
push yourself and keep
going. Competition
also gives you a sense
of achievement and a
natural high.

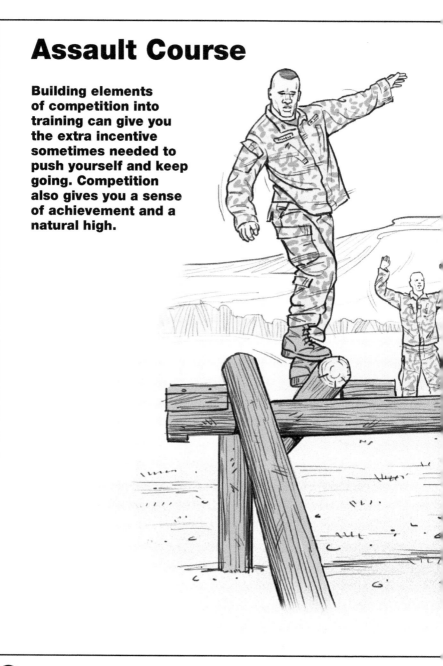

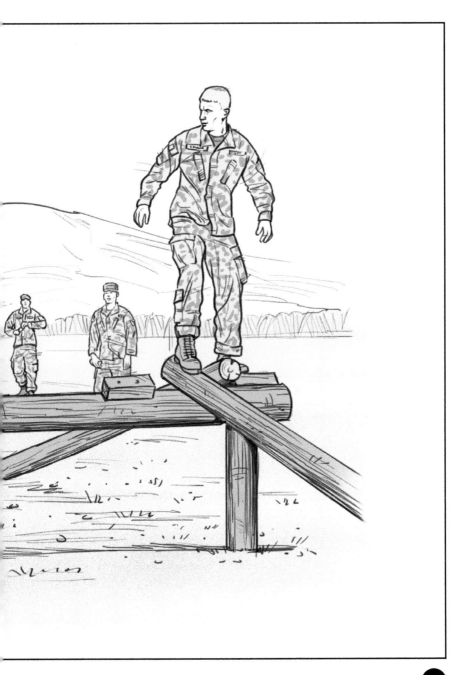

Surf Torture

The U.S. military regularly incorporates team building activities into training to build cooperation and motivation to succeed. This example of surf torture requires each person to work together and support one another under stressful and bitterly cold conditions.

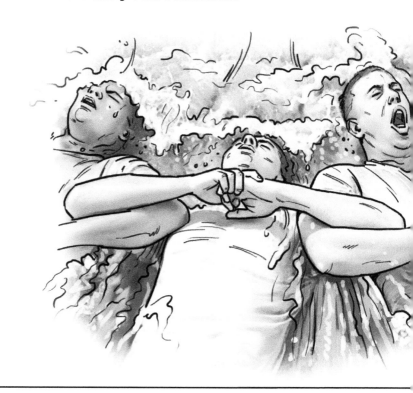

decide to drop out, to see if they have the mental grit to keep their focus on becoming a SEAL. The PTIs also want to see that the candidates work cooperatively.

Being a SEAL, indeed being a member of any elite unit, requires team-thinking at all times – the PTIs do not want to see someone purely focused on his own survival.

Following Hell Week and the remainder of Basic Conditioning comes the seven-week aquatic phase of the training – Combat

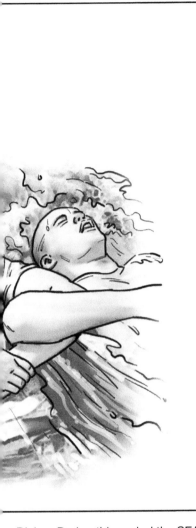

in stressful and often uncomfortable environments. Candidates who are 'not completely comfortable in the water often struggle to succeed' (U.S. Navy SEALs website). One infamous test is 'drown-proofing', in which the recruits have their wrists and ankles bound before being thrown into a swimming pool. (The hands are tied behind the back, just to make life doubly unpleasant.) Once in the pool, the candidates have to perform a range of exercises, all the while avoiding the real prospect of drowning:

- Bob up and down 20 times, propelling yourself off the bottom of the pool.
- Float for five minutes, using natural body buoyancy to prevent sinking.
- Swim to the shallow end of the pool, flip back without touching the bottom, then swim back to the other end of the pool.
- Do a forward and backward somersault underwater.
- Retrieve a snorkelling facemask from the bottom of the pool using the teeth.

Diving. During this period the SEALs are rarely out of the water. Not only will the candidates learn open- and closed-circuit diving techniques, the PTIs are also looking for those who 'demonstrate a high level of comfort in the water and the ability to perform

Drown-proofing is as much an exercise in suppressing panic as it is about lifesaving training. The PTIs are looking for people who can keep a clear head and focused actions, regardless of the environmental or psychological pressures.

Drown-proofing

This extreme activity helps test stress under pressure and builds self control and endurance, essential qualities for SEALs.

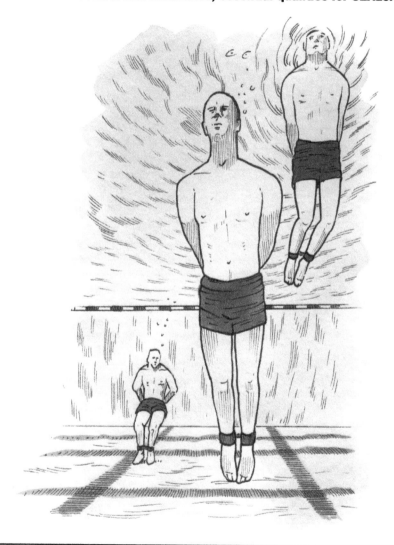

The Combat Diving programme introduces the candidates to all manner of underwater ordeals, including such horrors as swimming ashore on to rocks in rough sea and heavy waves, long-distance underwater swimming in low-visibility water and more tests of body-chilling endurance in the freezing surf. Those candidates who make it through this arduous phase then move on to seven weeks of Land Warfare Training (LWT) – teaching them infantry tactical and weapons skills – then the final stage, SEAL Qualification Training (SQT).

In SEAL Qualification Training, the few remaining candidates acquire the specialist military skills that will enable them to function in an active SEAL unit. The training includes: parachuting (both freefall and static line); Survival, Evasion, Resistance, Escape (SERE); cold-weather operations; combat first aid; amphibious warfare tactics; and air strike coordination. Both Land Warfare Training and Sea Warfare Training continue the physical ordeal of training, but these phases are more focused on the development of tactical skills and on testing the candidates' mental flexibility and creativity. Those who pass both these stages successfully receive the SEAL trident badge and are assigned to a SEAL unit, to begin their active service career in the Naval Special Forces.

'Irregular Exercise'

From the testimony of ex-SEALs, surviving BUD/S is primarily a matter of mental grit and resilience; physical fitness alone will not carry the candidate through such an exhausting regime. (More advice from ex-SEALs will be given in Chapter 7.) But the nature of BUD/S raises an important issue about physical conditioning for extreme fitness challenges. It is what I shall label 'irregular exercise', and it builds upon the points I made above about forging your physical development around contrasting exercise routines.

Many endurance sports involve regularity of movement. With marathon running events, for example, the main challenge is to keep placing one foot in front of the other, regardless of the undulations of the terrain or the number of hours you have been on the go. In a 10km (6-mile) swim, the swimmer needs to keep his chosen stroke going, repeating the action as efficiently as possible to power him through the water. Such challenges are true tests of human endurance, but they are essentially tests of repetitive movements. Athletes of these sports can struggle to perform, however, when they transfer to activities that feature broken sequences of awkward movements.

By way of proof, a recent British TV series – *SAS: Are You Tough Enough?* – featured ultra-fit members

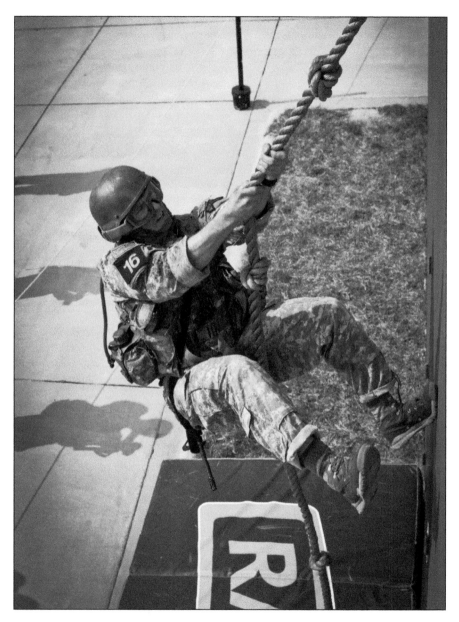

Military recruits need to be prepared for mental and physical challenges to be ready for live combat. Abseiling requires strength and self-belief.

Monkey Bars

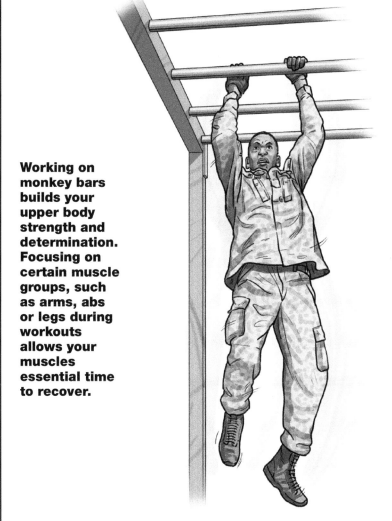

Working on
monkey bars
builds your
upper body
strength and
determination.
Focusing on
certain muscle
groups, such
as arms, abs
or legs during
workouts
allows your
muscles
essential time
to recover.

Training for Real Situations

Making someone combat-ready requires a great deal of self-determination, mental toughness and physical strength and endurance. Recruits must also prove their moral fibre, which is equally vital for deployment to war zones.

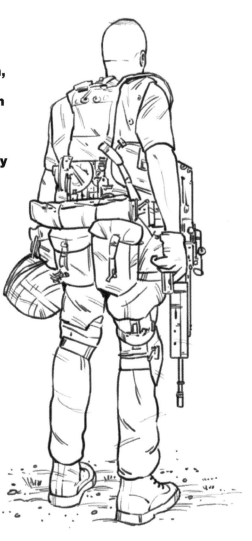

of the general public participating in a competition that replicated the selection procedure for the SAS. All participants came from strong extreme fitness backgrounds, competing in marathons, triathlons, iron man competitions and the like. The physical challenges were a formidable array of endurance tests mixed with mental challenges in tactical thinking. As with the real SAS selection course, few of the participants actually managed to complete the training course, despite the superb levels of physical conditioning they brought to the programme. Why?

From an observational point of view, a key reason was the introduction of various factors that broke the regularity of the exercise. For example, the contestants included people who could run for many kilometres on flat surfaces. Yet add a 25kg (55lb) rucksack to their bodies and send them up the undulating terrain of the Welsh mountains, and the drop-offs began. The weight of the pack affected the body's centre of balance, meaning that the core and upper-body muscles were having to work themselves constantly to keep the torso upright, adding to the steady depletion of energy. The landscape was both steep and perilous – tussocks of grass, boulders, holes in the ground and other obstacles meaning that it was hard to establish a regular

pace, and injuries such as twisted ankles or knees were a constant threat. The conditions imposed on the participants meant that all muscles of the body were in constant, erratic adjustment, and for many the unfamiliar, broken exercise – plus the weight addition provided by the pack – proved too much.

Inventive Exercise Programmes

What such programmes, and Special Forces training in general, demonstrate is the value of 'irregular exercise'. This is where we build irregular physical challenges into our exercise regime to improve all-round body conditioning and stamina. You can be as creative as you like. For example, a section of my typical hill run includes a pile of large rocks, each weighing several kilograms; carrying four or five of these (one at a time, of course) up a precipitous 50m (164ft) long section of muddy slope is, in many ways, far more exhausting than kilometres of regular running.

Similarly, think about ways in which you can adapt you own fitness routines to incorporate, on occasions, some irregular exercise activities that push you well out of your comfort zone. These can be as simple as carrying heavy, awkwardly shaped building materials around a convoluted physical space, or using training techniques such as a mud crawl to test your all-round fitness. Whatever you chose, make sure that

Under Fire

It is almost impossible to predict how you will react to extreme stresses such as being under fire. Here, the mental strength to keep going must be matched by the physical strength to do so, as doing nothing will likely result in capture or death.

it is safe to perform the exercise, and introduce the techniques gradually so that your body can adjust and reduce the chances of injury occurring.

Special Forces training provides us with some additional inspiration for developing irregular exercise techniques. The British Royal Marines are a case in point. Passing through the Royal Marines selection process, then maintaining the standards of fitness required by 3 Commando

Brigade Royal Marines, is not for the faint-hearted. Commando training lasts 32 weeks for enlisted men, and 64 weeks for officers, and attrition is above 75 per cent. The Royal Marines are the armed services experts in cold-weather warfare, and training includes immersion in icy holes in frozen lakes in arctic Norway, from which the recruit has to claw his way out (while wearing his pack) using only his ski sticks and body weight.

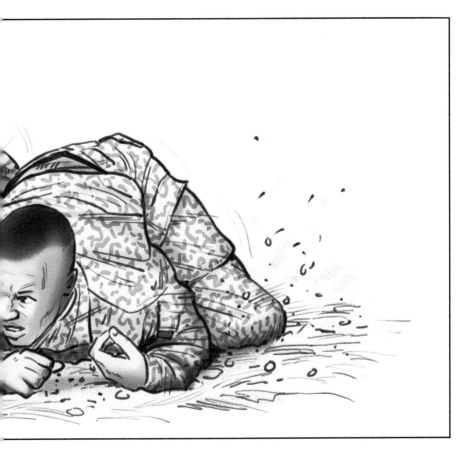

The Royal Marines have pioneered their own set of tests to evaluate both the recruits in training and the soldiers under their command. Some of these are written down in the 2011 publication *Royal Marine Fitness Tests* (available online at www.royalnavy.mod.uk/custom/navy/trainingtool.html), and they can be useful to civilians wanting to build variety into their own extreme fitness development.

An initial example is the Royal Marines' Representative Military Tests (RM RMT), which are 'designed to assess their troops' speed, endurance and muscular strength through a series of aerobic activities, which may be used in conjunction with other RM physical tests or role-related training. Note that these tests are not performed in PT gear; instead they are carried out in full CS95 combat uniform, boots, load-

Serial (a)	Test (b)	Conditions (c)	Rationale (d)
1.	Fireman's carry of 100m (328ft) on good terrain	Weapon slung and in a time of 45 seconds, partner of similar size/weight	Simulated casualty evacuation. Functional test of upper and lower body strength
2.	Perform $1/2$ regain on single rope	Rope height to be minimum 2.25m (7ft 4in), weapon slung	Functional test of combat agility and upper body strength
3.	Carry 2 x 20kg (44lb) jerry cans 150m (492ft)	Weapon slung	Fuel/water resupply and approx weight of a two-man stretcher carry with casualty
4.	Shuttle sprints – 5 x 20m (65ft) in 56 seconds	Carrying weapon b. Adopting a prone position at the 20, 40, 60 and 80m (65, 131, 196 and 262ft) marks	Functional test of anaerobic muscular endurance using a simulated section attack
5.	Climb and descend a 9.14m (30ft) rope	Weapon slung, correct climbing technique	Functional test of combat agility and upper body strength

– Royal Marines, *Royal Marine Fitness Tests*, p.63

carrying equipment and weapon (an SA80 assault rifle), the total combined weight of kit being 13.22kg (29lb). The tests are featured in the table above.

The activities described here perfectly embody the principles of irregular exercise outlined above. Note how the challenges are tied to actual trials that could face the soldier in the combat arena, such as carrying a stretcher or casualty across a battlefield. Multi-physical aspects of the soldier's physique are tested, including upper-body strength, lower-body strength, anaerobic fitness and aerobic endurance. At the same time as performing the challenge, the recruit must negotiate the awkward loads presented by his own kit and slung weapon, with heavy straps reducing circulation to limbs and therefore increasing fatigue.

Ice Climbing

The endurance required to tackle this ice sheet is made more difficult by facing the extremes of cold weather. Frigid air means it is harder to take in oxygen, making this physical feat even more challenging.

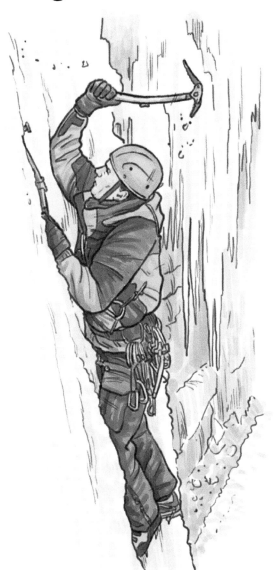

Stretcher Race

Military training aims to be as close as possible to life in the field. Stretcher races test teamwork, endurance and speed under pressure.

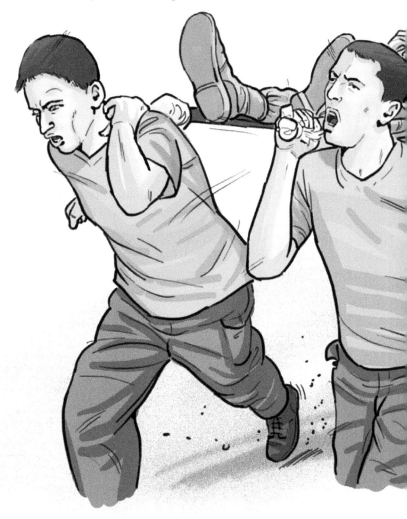

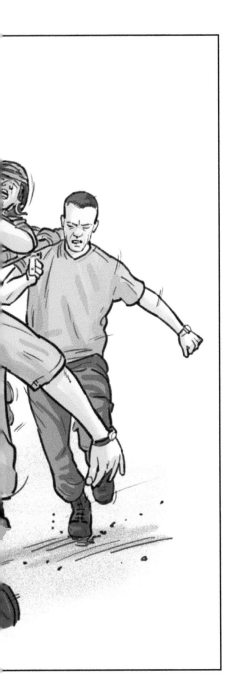

Many of these exercises can be replicated in your fitness programme, especially if you have a good training partner. Indeed, partner training adds many fresh opportunities within your fitness routines. You can practice, for example, performing endurance runs while carrying long sections of heavy pipe between you on your shoulders, or alternating carrying heavy weights such as water-filled jerry cans. Individually, you can also soup-up your training by adding military-style uniform and kit to your training regime, such as belt weights and a backpack, and carrying an item roughly along the same length and weight as a rifle. Anything that essentially adds new demands on your physiology will enhance your training. Once again, this advice comes with the caution against introducing anything too extreme in the first instance. Irregular exercise often carries with it increased risks in injury, especially to knee and ankle joints and to the back muscles, so make sure that you acclimatize to the new forms of training.

Lessons from the Elite

In the remainder of this chapter, we shall peek inside the training regimes of other elite forces to see what forms of exercise they use, and how they can be applied to non-military settings. Looking once again at the Royal Marines, recruits must eventually perform four

High Wall

Obstacle courses build cooperation while utilizing varied muscle groups.

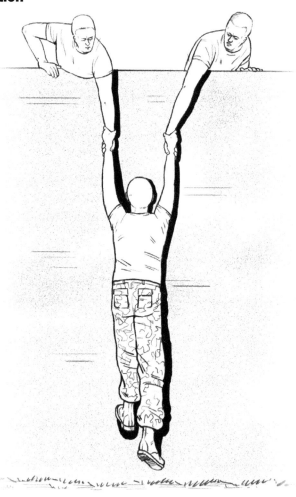

'commando tests' towards the end of their training, each test a punishing endurance test in its own right. The RM website describes the four tests as follows:

- **The endurance course** – *you will work your way through 3.2km (2 miles) of tunnels, pools, streams, bogs and woods, then run 6.4km (4 miles) back to camp, all while you're in combat equipment and carrying a weapon, and all in less than 72 minutes. When you get back, you'll have to get six out of ten shots on target in a shooting test.*
- **The 14.4km (9 mile) speed march** – *you need to complete this in 90 minutes while carrying your equipment and a rifle.*
- **The Tarzan assault course** – *an aerial slide, ropes course, assault course and 9.1m (30ft) wall, which you will need to complete in 13 minutes, while carrying your equipment and a rifle.*
- **The (48.2km (30 mile) march** – *a 48.2km (30 mile) march across Dartmoor, which you will need to complete in under eight hours with your equipment and a rifle. Officers must cover the same route in seven hours.*

– www.royalnavy.mod.uk/Careers/ Royal-Marines/How-To-Join-the-Marines/RM-Commando-Training

The four tests alternate roughly between endurance runs and obstacle-course events, and each includes elements of mental testing as well as physical challenge. The endurance course, for example, includes a totally water-filled tunnel through which the recruit must crawl, in full kit, while already out of breath from previous challenges. The Tarzan assault course is a trial of nerve, the candidate having to tackle each obstacle with commitment, despite the threat of injuries from falls and impact.

The military are lovers of obstacle courses in general, and it is not hard to understand why. Obstacles courses are uniquely energy sapping, testing every major muscle group with challenges such as rope swings and climbs, log runs, tyre runs, climbing walls and crawl pits. By being fixed training facilities, obstacle courses encourage a competitive spirit as each class attempts to achieve the best overall time. Furthermore, some obstacles can only be tackled by team effort, thus they encourage a spirit of cooperation.

Others test pure nerve. A good example of this type of course is the British Parachute Regiment's 'Trainasium' – an 'aerial confidence course' set 17m (55ft) above the ground. Without any safety net, the candidate has to perform series of jumps between separate platforms over dizzying drops, with the

Teamwork

Impossible individual feats can be achieved through teamwork.

Difficult Terrain

Covering terrains such as streams or mud can be physically exhausting. They require extreme self-control and the will to survive.

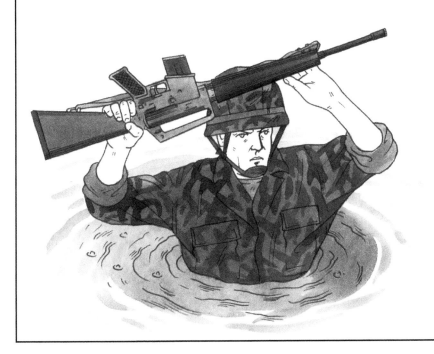

unforgiving trainers looking for any hesitation or loss of nerve.

Obstacle courses are undoubtedly good ways in which to develop the adaptable physique and competitive spirit needed for extreme fitness development. They also have the benefit of exposing those who don't have the team mentality. This revelation could be especially important if you are planning on a team extreme fitness challenge – better to find out on an assault course that you can't work with someone rather than out in the wilderness somewhere.

With some research, you should be able to find good assault course facilities within easy travelling distance. Check out websites first.

Ranger School Exercises

The following are physical training exercises recommended by the U.S. Army Ranger School:

Floor wiper – using a barbell loaded with the prescribed weight, lie on your back and press the weight up as if you were bench-pressing it. Keep the arms locked out, and lift your legs up together and touch the left plate. Lower your legs down to the floor then lift them back up to the right plate. Repeat.

KB figure 8 – kettlebell figure eight. Hold a kettlebell at the prescribed weight in one hand. Pass the KB from hand to hand and in between your legs in a figure eight pattern.

Medicine ball toss and run – with a 9kg (20lb) medicine ball, throw the ball as far as you can, chase after it and repeat.

Wall ball – stand with the feet shoulder width apart facing a wall. Hold a 9kg (20lb) ball under your chin, squat to parallel and explode up to the standing position. As you reach the standing position push/throw the ball up to a 3m (10ft) target. Catch the ball and repeat.

Depth jump – stand on a platform approx 46cm (18in) high. Jump off the platform and when your feet hit the ground drop into a full squat, then jump out of the squat as high as you can.

Get up – holding the prescribed weight in one hand at shoulder level, lay flat on the ground. Then, stand or 'get up' to you feet. Lay back down on your back (holding the weight at shoulder level the entire time) and repeat.

Thruster – hold a barbell in the rack position (on the top of your shoulders) with your hands approximately shoulder width apart. Squat to parallel and explode up to the standing position. As you reach the standing position the bar should continue to travel to overhead. Lower the bar back to the rack position and repeat.

– U.S. Army Rangers, *Range School Preparation*, p.6

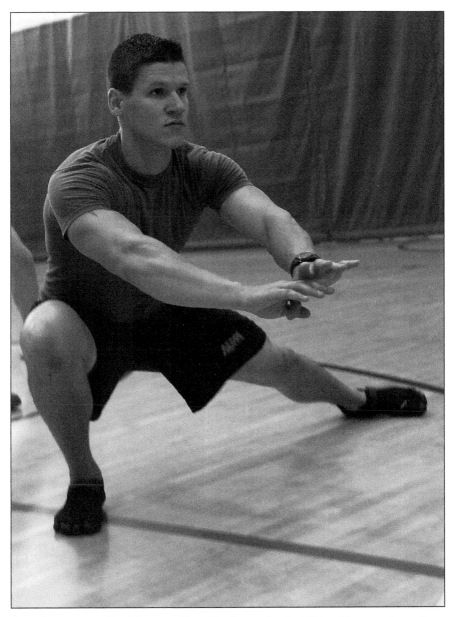

Squats are excellent for working the lower body. This side squat works the gluts, hamstrings and calves. Perform such exercises on both sides.

Helicopter Rescue

Special Forces training intensifies in difficulty and danger as it progresses. A helicopter rescue requires high levels of teamwork, courage and upper-body strength.

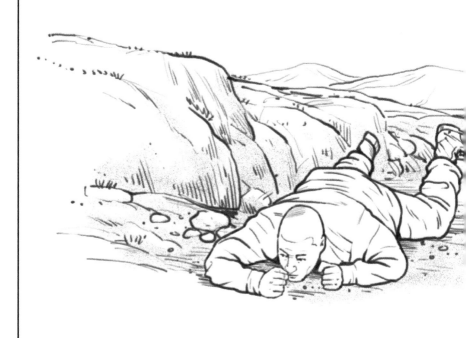

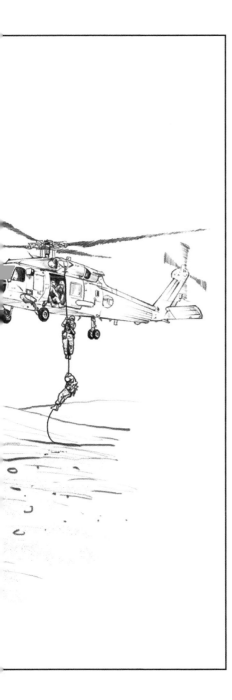

The obstacles should present a balanced mix of challenges to develop endurance, strength, cardio-fitness, core training and flexibility, and check whether they can be configured for different levels of fitness. You should ensure that the company has properly safety standards for its equipment, and also that qualified trainers are on hand to guide you through every aspect of the course. Avoid courses where too many people are allowed to go around at any one time – a maximum of eight is a good number.

Boot Camp and SERE Training

In addition to military-style obstacle courses, there are also many ex-military personnel offering 'boot camp'-style training sessions. The nature of these boot camps varies enormously, from light cardiovascular exercise for weight loss through to Special Forces intensity training only intended for the super fit. Some even include elements such as SERE (Survive, Evade, Resist, Extract) training for those who wish to test their minds as well as their bodies. In SAS training, the four-week SERE element comes fairly late in the selection process. By the time the candidate reaches this stage he will have survived nearly four months of physical and mental punishment. The ordeals suffered during the initial 'Endurance' phase of training are

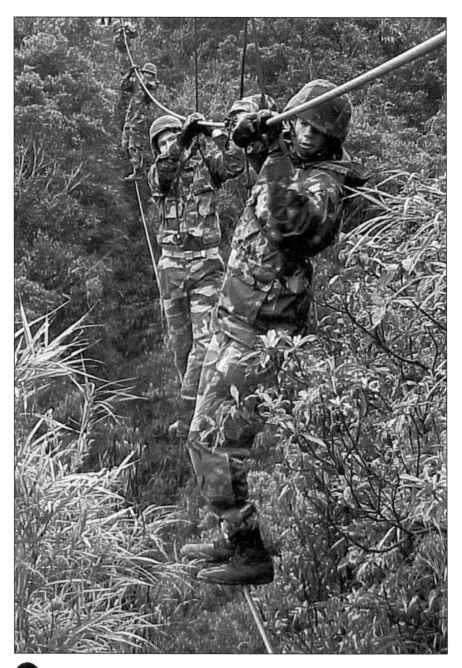

Opposite: Rope walking requires nerve, balance and technique. With several men on the rope, one person losing their balance could knock everyone off.

legendary. They culminate in the 'Long Drag', a sub-20 hour, 64km (40 mile) march over the Brecon Beacons mountain wearing 25kg (55lb) of kit, all while performing complex navigational tasks.

By the time the Endurance phase ends, about 60 per cent of the class will have dropped out. This phase is followed by four weeks of 'Continuation Training' – small-unit tactics and advanced combat skills, before the candidates spend six weeks learning survival and tactical skills in the rainforests of Borneo.

Then, if the candidate is still in the running he goes on four weeks of SERE. Here he is further trained in the skills of wilderness survival, and also in how to both evade capture and survive interrogation if he does fall into enemy hands. The training is extremely realistic, with the candidate being pursued across kilometres of countryside by a dedicated tracking force with modern technology. Most individuals are eventually captured, and then subjected to moderated forms of physical and mental torture (such as sleep deprivation and being forced to stand for long periods in stress positions) in an attempt to get them to divulge information.

The entire SERE course requires strong nerves to complete successfully, and it might seem surprising that some people would do it willingly. Nevertheless, courses are provided by private companies, mostly for civilians or military contractors going into high-risk situations, but also for those of an adventurous spirit.

SERE training can undoubtedly add a new and highly unusual element to your civilian fitness programme, if you have the time, money and the inclination. You will have to cover long distances on foot, while constantly exercising your intelligence with the problems of detection and evasion.

If caught, your physical stamina will help you through some of the stress position ordeals, while hardening your mental control. Yet do remember that survival training is not necessarily a form of extreme fitness training per se (although it is undoubtedly a good skill set to have for wilderness events).

Survival is often more about energy conservation than energy expenditure, and matching your physical activity with a greatly reduced calorie intake. Nevertheless, like many aspects of elite forces training, Survival, Evasion, Resistance, Escape offers a way to test body and mind to the limit, while also acquiring a survival knowledge that may have later applications.

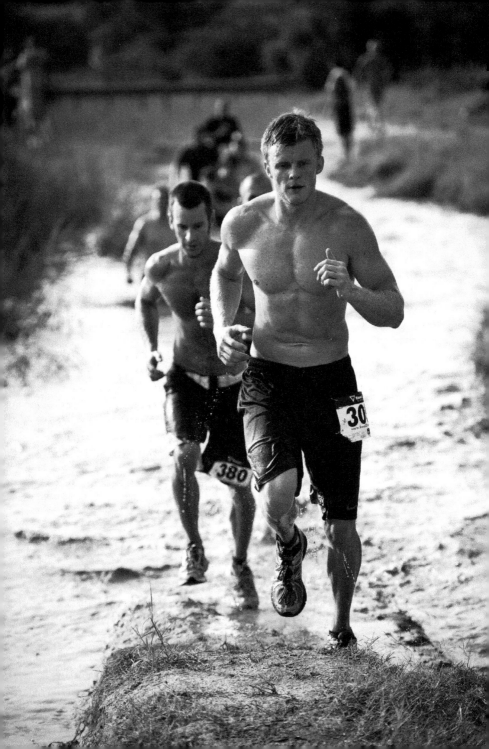

Any soldier who attempts to join the Special Forces, and succeeds, will become intimately acquainted with the capabilities of his own legs. Running, or at least fast marching, constitutes a large part of the military training, for the simple reason that the soldier's legs will often be his or her primary means of deployment on the battlefield. What makes the soldier's experience very much different from the typical civilian runner is that he will have to carry heavy loads at the same time.

During the Falklands War in 1982, the British lost most of their heavy-lift Chinook helicopters when the transport vessel Atlantic Conveyor was hit and sunk by an Exocet missile. This meant that many of the soldiers on land had no means of deployment other than walking, hence men of the Parachute Regiment and Royal Marines 'yomped' 90km (56 miles) in three days, through terrible weather across treacherous terrain. To add to their burden, each man carried 36kg (80lb) of pack, ammunition and weaponry.

Pushing to the Limit

Running's popularity is very easy to understand. Running is a very accessible sport, requiring limited kit and minimal training – an amateur

....

Opposite: Extreme running is a superb way of developing overall fitness and strength.

3

Running is by far the most popular extreme fitness event. The permutations of this sport are tremendously varied, and range from straightforward road runs through to distance ordeals in some of the world's most perilous climates.

Extreme Running

Long-Distance Racing

When running in large groups, set your own pace, not that of the people around you. Many people set off too quickly, buoyed by the adrenaline of the race, but find they can't sustain the pace in the long run.

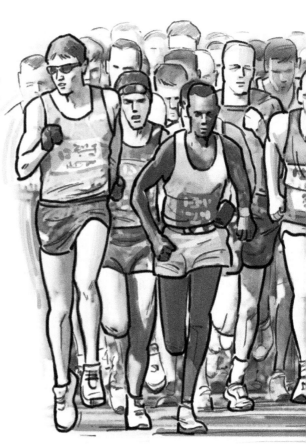

runner can simply pull on a pair of decent trainers and some basic running clothes, and head out from his front door. Running also provides undeniable health benefits. These include:

- Fat-burning (c. 400 calories burnt in 30 minutes running)
- Reduce the chances of osteoporosis in later life
- Improved cardiovascular health
- Reduces the risk of developing

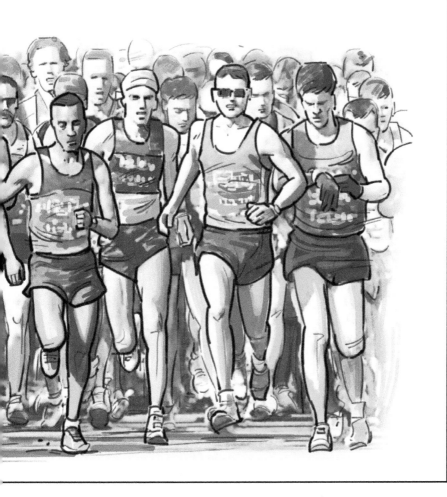

dementia in later life
- Positive effect on mental health via reduced stress levels.

The range of running challenges can also suit every level of personal fitness. For unfit people entirely new to running, a 5k (3.1 mile) race might be the ultimate, and achievable, goal. For those with greater ambitions and matching levels of stamina, a 42km (26 mile) marathon is a classic option.

(At the time of writing, the current world marathon record is just 2.03:38, an astonishing time set by the Kenyan runner Patrick Makau.) But there are extreme fitness challenges for the running community that put even marathons in the shade. These events typically involve multiple marathon-lengths runs over consecutive days, and often through terrain and weather that would make walking alone exhausting. A few of the big international events are:

Marathon de Sable – this epic six-day race covers 251km (156 miles) of the Sahara desert in southern Morocco in temperatures that often exceed 40°C (104°F).

Grand to Grand Ultra – a winding 237km (147 miles) route through the Utah desert, the Grand to Grand Ultra is a seven-day race relying on the athletes carrying their own means of life support. The terrain ascends to elevations of 5791m (19,000ft).

Jungle Ultra – a 229.5km (142.6 mile) run through precipitous Peruvian jungle, the self-supported Jungle Ultra race pits the runner against tropical temperatures, energy-sapping humidity, dangerous wildlife and truly ankle-snapping terrain.

Badwater Ultra-marathon – this non-stop 217km (135 mile) race through Death Valley, the hottest place on Earth, during July – the hottest month of the year – includes crossing two mountain ranges.

These extraordinary races, and others, are almost unsurpassed tests of mind and body. Because of the load-carrying and tactical aspects of their physical challenges, the Special Forces community rarely covers such distances during their training and selection programmes, but they do explore the limits of human endurance on two feet.

A case in point is the SAS selection runs/marches. When the SAS recruit arrives for training at their headquarters, he is treated to the usual battery of initial fitness assessments, such as basic distance runs against fixed times. The initial week of induction is just a prelude to a hyper-demanding four weeks of endurance and navigation training. The most revered aspects of this phase are the 'Fan Dance' and the 'Long Drag'. True to its name, the 'Fan Dance' relates to the mountain of Pen y Fan, 886m (2907ft) high in the Brecon Beacons mountain range in South Wales. Essentially the Fan Dance is a 24km (15 mile) endurance march repeatedly up and down this most precipitous of landscapes, all the while navigating accurately between features and carrying 15kg (33lb) of pack plus rifle. Those who complete this challenge successfully go on to tackle the Long Drag – 64km

Running with Pack

When running with a pack, ensure that it is adjusted as close to your centre of gravity as possible. Lean forward to take weight off the straps and shorten the length of your stride.

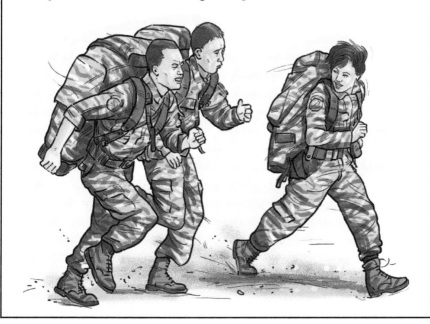

(40 miles) in 20 hours, with 25kg (55lb) backpack and rifle.

Needless to say, many people are beaten by these extreme physical challenges. The endurance phase is conducted in both winter and high summer, the season bringing its own individual problems for the recruits. Indeed, at the time of writing the SAS has been much-publicized for the deaths of no fewer than three recruits who died of hyperthermia (heatstroke) suffered when attempting to complete an endurance march during an exceptionally hot day. Such utter tragedies indicate the level of physical pressure exerted on all who attempt to join the SAS – all the men who died were serving territorial or regular army soldiers, some of whom had experienced tours of Afghanistan.

Elite forces training places similar demands to the ultra-marathons described above. They require that the individual maintain a regular pace of run or fast walk over many hours, relying on cardiovascular resources, muscle strength and sheer mental will power to keep him going. How to achieve such levels of endurance is the topic of this chapter.

Mechanics

Before going on to look at how to train and conduct extreme running events, we need to probe a little more closely into the topic of running itself. People have always run – references to endurance runners can be found back in Classical antiquity – but it is only in the last few decades that the physical mechanics of running has been scientifically unpacked and understood. This has provided trainers with data and information about the optimal running form.

A run differs from a fast walk in that while running you spend a brief moment when both feet are off the ground. (With a walk, there is always one foot in contact with the floor at any one time.) While this basic action is what all people who run have in common, there is great variation in the styles of running, with equal variation in terms of efficiency. Let's now look at the core principles of a good running style, then we can address things that you might be doing wrong. A treadmill and a mirror

(or someone to film you) are near-essential tools for refining your style, unless you can go running with a colleague who has an eye trained for such matters.

The key points of an efficient endurance running style are:

- Keep your upper torso straight, although leaning forward slightly, and the back of the neck should be aligned naturally upwards. Don't hunch your back (which interferes with natural hip extension) or bend your neck forward (which can result in a strain injury).
- Push off the foot with your toe, allowing the foot to roll forward naturally when applying power. Push forward, rather than up, for maximum speed efficiency.
- Through the stride, keep your arms held at a 90-degree angle at the elbow. Swing them in straight lines backwards and forwards, from the shoulders rather than from the elbows. Don't hold your arms either too high or too low, as both positions induce strain, and don't let your arms cross your body's frontal centreline.
- When your foot lands, the knee should be slightly bent. The calf should be about perpendicular with the ground, and the point of impact should actually be close to the body's centreline,

Running Technique

When running, lean slightly forward with the torso, keep your head up, and swing your arms as if they are on rails by the side of your body.

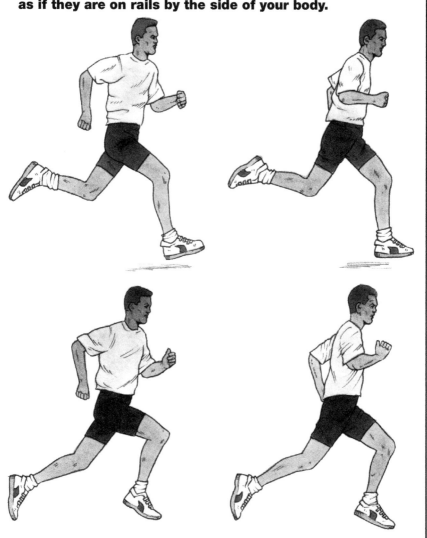

Quad Presses

Great for developing quad muscles, quad presses also strengthen the muscles supporting the knee. This can prevent running injuries, such as the varieties of 'runner's knee'.

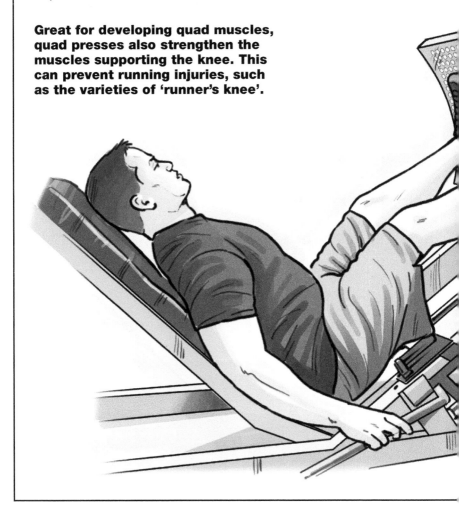

striking more with your midstep. Don't adopt a long stride in which you strike with your heel well ahead of your body, as this is both inefficient and more liable to induce impact injuries.

- For endurance running, try not to lift the knee too much; a high knee lift is more characteristic of sprinting.

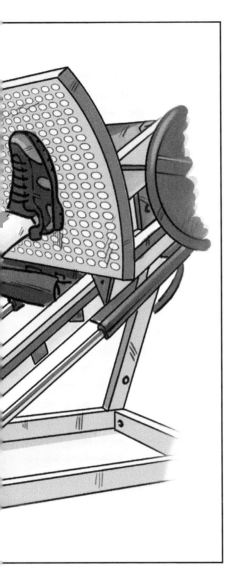

For those with the available time and money, special running assessment centres are available in many high-quality sports centres. By monitoring your run on a treadmill, the

instructors can coach you out of the bad habits many of us pick up, and revitalize your running method and times. For reference, here are some of the common mistakes runners can make in their technique:

Heavy impact – avoid a technique that inflicts a heavy impact on your heel with every stride, which can eventually result in a range of painful stress injuries. Don't push your leg out too far in front of you (note the point above about keeping the point of impact close to the centreline) and be conscious of placing your foot on the ground, rather than striking the ground.

Limited movement – the opposite problem to that described previously, here the runner has only a very small range of movement in both the arms and the legs, producing a shuffling gait. Although the physical impact levels are low, ironically it can still produce injuries over time, including shin splints and knee problems. Lift your heels to compensate, and feel that you are cycling the leg from your thigh and buttocks, rather than just from the knee.

Upward movement – avoid high vertical bounces in your running technique. Not only will these heighten the risk of impact injuries, they will also slow your times substantially – you are meant to be travelling forward, not upward. Pump your arms more quickly to force your legs into a better rhythm, and focus on pushing forward along the ground rather than bouncing off it.

Erratic arms – your arms have a key relationship to your run, their rhythm and regularity mirroring that of your stride. Moreover, by pumping the arms faster the torsional effect on your upper body results in an increase of pace. Losing control of your arms therefore has a detrimental effect on your running speed, as well as putting strain on your lower back and hips. Arms often become desynchronized with the legs when the runner gets tired during a long race, with the arms circling independently of the legs. Keep a conscious focus on maintaining a rhythmic arm movement, with the arms in the correct position. Invest in upper-body strengthening exercises to ensure that you have the muscular strength to maintain arm posture for the duration of a race. Also be careful not to let you arms swing across your body's centreline. Practice keeping the arms swinging by the side of the body – you can check this by standing in front of a mirror and looking at the swing of your arms.

Work on your core technique diligently, as it is the foundation of any running event. You can also improve your running speed and endurance by cross-training.

Swimming and cycling, for example, will have a positive impact on your endurance levels, as alongside your running they will help develop a well-rounded physique, less prone to fatigue. Targeted weight training is very beneficial. Focus on exercises that will improve the strength of the shoulders, abdominal muscles, lower back and buttocks, while leg press and leg extension reps will provide some extra power to the lower limbs.

Equipment

The Running Shoe

Running equipment is one area where science has rather overcomplicated matters. For the new runner, the choice of footwear in particular has become a matter of vast and bewildering choice. Here I can provide some recommendations, but there is no substitute for the personal advice of a running expert in a good sports shop. The best outlets will have treadmills in the store so the staff can observe your running technique and provide you with the right shoe.

Your first selection criterion for a running shoe is to decide what type of running you actually want to do. If you intend to do most of your running on tracks, tarmac or similar flat surface, you will need a shoe with a decent degree of cushioning and, possibly, motion control built into the structure to reduce the chance

Running Shoes

Different surfaces
require different levels
of grip. Here we see
trail shoes (top) plus
trainers with ice grips
fitted over the sole.

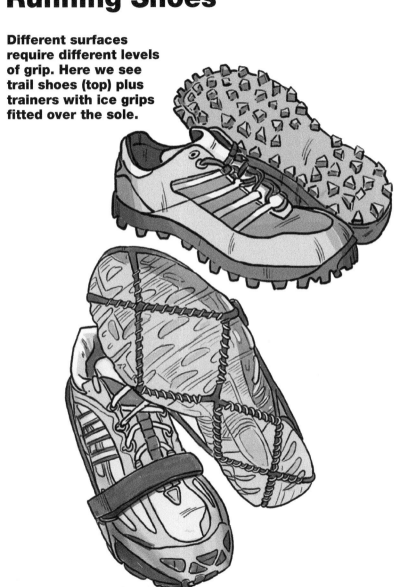

Shoe versus Barefoot Running

While the shoe offers protection against objects and cushions impact, barefoot running can be very efficient and helps mimimize heel strike injuries. Note the cushioning bent knee of the landing leg in the figure on the left, as opposed to the shoed runer below.

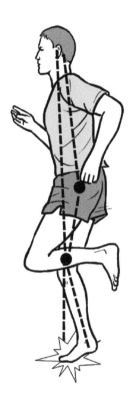

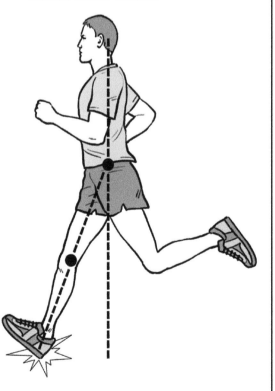

of injury from repeated pounding on a hard surface. If, by contrast, you intend to run mostly off-road, you need a trail shoe, which is stiffer, has a more neutral balance (the foot is more mobile on uneven surfaces) and, crucially, improved grip on the sole, good enough to achieve adhesion on grass and mud.

As we make more subtle distinctions between footware, we can divide the shoes into the following categories:

Motion control – these shoes are designed to correct over pronation (when the feet roll too much inward as the pressure transfers from the heel to the toes). They have features built into the sole to control the excessive movement, and tend to be quite rigid in structure. Many larger runners find a motion-control shoe practical.

Neutral cushioned – cushioned running shoes, as their name suggests, provide plenty of cushioning to the foot to protect it from impact. This type of shoe has cushioning centred around the midsole and minimum arch support, and therefore suit those whose feet work in a biomechanically efficient manner, with high or normal arches.

Stability – good for those with low to normal arches, and who have moderate overpronation. Stability shoes provide support across the range of foot impact, including for the midsole.

Performance – performance shoes are ultra light and are designed for committed racers. They come with a variety of advanced stability features.

Minimalist – these have limited cushioning and suit the biomechanically efficient runner who wants a lot of responsiveness from his shoe, often when running off-road events. Those who use this type of shoe need a good, low-impact style if they are to avoid injuries.

Barefoot – the barefoot shoe essentially just provides the foot with protection from foreign objects; it provides almost no cushioning whatsoever. Barefoot shoes are for those who subscribe to the practice of barefoot running (running in a way that reflects how we would run barefoot) and for those who want to strengthen their lower-limb muscles.

Even with these categories to guide us, the matter of buying the right trainer is primarily a case of trying out different brands and styles until you find one that suits you. Here are some quick tips to help you with the buying process:

1. Don't buy shoes that are too tight, as your feet will swell up while running. Try them on in

the afternoon (when your feet have already become larger) and while wearing your choice of running socks.

2. Try the shoes out on the shop treadmill – just walking around the store itself isn't a good enough test.

3. Don't necessarily go for the most attractive fashion brands; rather, only buy shoes that protect your feet and will enhance your run.

4. Know when to buy. You should aim to change your running shoes about every 800km (500 miles) of running. If you start to feel your knees, ankles or back aching after a run, it could be that your shoes need replacing.

Clothing

Running clothing needn't be extravagant, although for extreme fitness events – where you might be running for many hours or even days – it pays to invest in good kit. For your feet, high-quality running socks are the natural choice. Not only do they incorporate their own cushioning features that reduce the likelihood of blisters, they also have enhanced elasticated support for the whole foot, no toe seams to catch on nails and breathable fabric that helps with sweat release. On your lower body you can wear either shorts or running tights. Either way, they should have a comfortable elasticated waistband, a small zipped pocket for holding those essential items such as keys or money and ideally some fluorescent features to keep you visible in low-light conditions. Your T-shirt should be brightly coloured with non-chafing flatback seams. The fabric should have a UV coating to protect you from the sun, and made of a 'breathable' material that wicks away sweat.

For running in cooler and wetter conditions, a running jacket is an essential addition. Like the T-shirt, it should be fully breathable but also waterproof and windproof to stop you getting soaked to the skin on inclement runs; vents in strategic locations will also help with sweat release and air circulation. Adjustable waistbands and cuffs give you a degree of comfort and temperature control. Ensure that the jacket is snug fitting, but is designed for flexible movement – it must really feel like a second skin when you are wearing it, and no parts of it should chafe. (A key point to remember with running kit is that a niggling rub over 5km/3.1 miles could turn into an agonizing open sore over 20–30km/12–18 miles.) A lightweight, breathable UV-treated running cap is also a good idea for protecting the face from both rain and sun.

For women, a sports bra is essential to prevent ligament damage to the breasts. A good sports bra should limit movement by at least

U.S. Army Advice on Purchasing a Running Shoe

When shopping for running shoes, keep the following in mind:

- Expect to spend between $50 and $150 for a pair of good shoes.
- Discuss your foot type, foot problems and shoe needs with a knowledgeable salesperson.
- Check the PX [post exchange] for available brands and their prices before shopping at other stores.
- Buy a training shoe, not a racing shoe.
- When trying on shoes, wear socks that are as similar as possible to those in which you will run.

Also, be sure to try on both shoes, and look at more than one model of shoe.

- Choose a pair of shoes that fit both feet well while you are standing.
- Ask if you can try running in the shoes on a non-carpeted surface. This gives you a feel for the shoes.
- Carefully inspect the shoes for defects that might have been missed by quality control. Do the following:
  – Place the shoes on a flat surface and check the heel from behind to see that the heel cup is perpendicular to the sole of the shoe.
  – Feel the seams inside the shoe to determine if they are smooth, even and well-stitched.
  – Check for loose threads or extra glue spots; they are usually signs of poor construction.

  – U.S. Army, FM 21-20, Appendix E

Running Gear

Comfort and ease of movement are key when choosing running gear. If you need to carry anything, chose clothing with zippable pockets. Here we see running shorts, breathable/waterproof jacket and T-shirt, plus water-carrying belt, runner's backpack and training shoes. GPS watches are a handy addition for performance and distance monitoring.

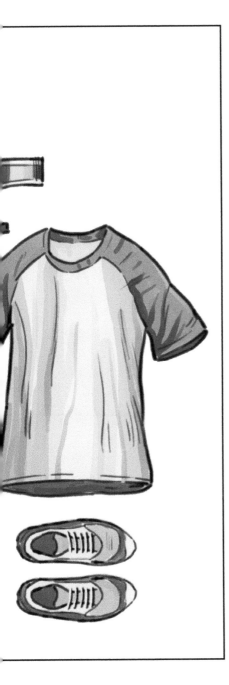

60 per cent, with cups that fully encase each breast and straps with no more than 2.5cm (1in) of give. Make sure that the underband does not chafe or rub. If possible, have your bra professionally fitted to ensure that it is exactly the right size.

Useful Kit

For extreme running there is a plethora of other types of gear available to support your running efforts. While space limits what we can list and describe, here are some key items many professional distance runners now find useful.

Running/GPS watch – a basic running watch will tell you how far you have run and your average pace, and will include an internal data log so you can keep track of your run data. Spend larger amounts of money, however, and features can include a heart rate monitor (via a wireless chest band), GPS distance monitoring and navigation, altitude counter, training zone monitor, pace indicators and wirelessly transferred data log.

Water carrier – although many races provide water stations, for training or endurance runs carrying your own fluid is essential. For small amounts of fluid (250–500ml/0.4–0.9 pints), a fist-grip bottle is a practical hand-held option. Practice running while holding this bottle before you begin a race; the extra weight can affect your

GPS and Trail Running Pack

Running packs can hold everything you need for a trail run, as well as carrying weights if you choose to load it. A GPS watch is useful to monitor your run data and plan progression.

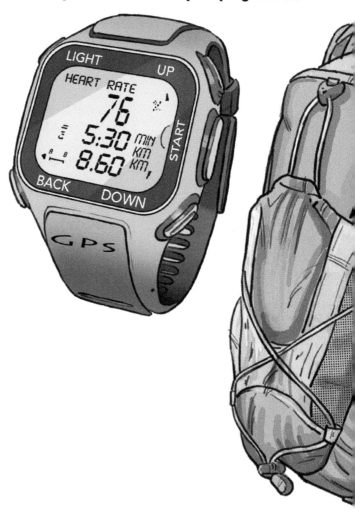

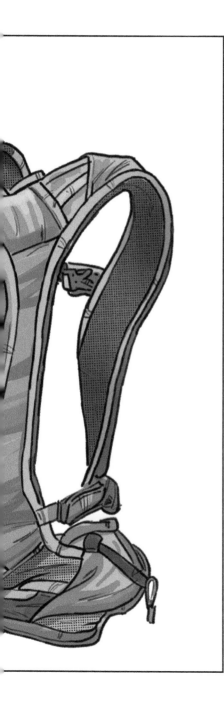

balance and arm swing if you are not used to it. An option for greater distances is to carry multiple water bottles in a belt carrier, or to adopt a high-capacity hydration pack. The latter can be either a belt pack or even a backpack style bladder (Camelbak are a leading brand), with several litres of fluid available to drink on the run through a tube. The weight of water packs can be substantial, so ensure that they are fitted snugly and do not rub even after many kilometres of running.

Running backpack – for self-sufficient endurance runs, particularly through extreme terrain, a running backpack is essential. Buy one that is big enough to handle everything you need for an event – they can range in size from diminutive 10-litre (17.5-pint) models up to huge backpacks with more than 30 litres (53 pints) capacity. The backpack should have fully adjustable shoulder, waist and chest straps to restrict the pack's movement while running, and the fabric needs to be waterproof and breathable (breathability helps reduce uncomfortable sweat build-up between your back and the pack fabric). It also needs plenty of pouches to store individual items, and can include a hydration reservoir and drinking tube system.

Camping equipment – for overnight self-sufficient runs in the wilderness,

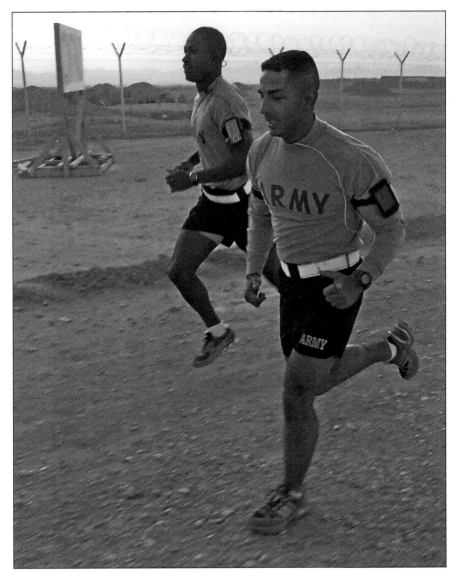

Above: Listening to music while you run can help you get into a step rhythm and maintain your focus and energy levels for longer.

a basic shelter is requisite. You can either go for a lightweight tent plus a sleeping bag, or a sleeping bag with a waterproof bivvy bag cover. The latter combination is probably best for one or two nights in the wild at most, and in fairly forgiving weather conditions, but for more adverse climates and multi-day challenges a tent is the best option. The range of options and technologies for tents is vast, so your best bet is to visit a professional camping or endurance running shop and get them to provide something exactly modelled to your needs.

Distance Runs

Preparation is essential if you plan to take on any extreme distance run. Much obviously depends upon your current status as a runner. If your longest distance run has been a 5km (3.1 miles), and you intend to tackle a marathon, then you have much work to do. Yet even a very seasoned distance runner should invest in a conscious plan of development when intending to take on any extreme fitness challenge.

If you are new to long-distance running, then a graduated scheme of exercise is critical. Work up your distances progressively and mix your running styles to suit your fitness levels. Your first objective is to build up endurance. Run initially for time, not distance, focusing on establishing a good pace for a fixed duration. Once your body is comfortable with running for a certain period, you can increase either the length of time run or the distance you attempt to run within a time. A mixture of both

strategies is good to improve both speed and endurance.

When building up to doing a marathon, your running week will naturally incorporate plenty of distance runs, increasing the distance on a weekly basis. With commitment, a runner with minimal distance running experience can build up to a marathon standard in 16 weeks, with weekly distances beginning at around 40km (25 miles) and reaching up to 50km (31 miles) in the pre-race week. Keep a meticulous running log, detailing each run in terms of time/distance, the time of day you did the run, the terrain covered and even factors such as the weather and how often you rehydrated. By including as much detail as possible in your running log, you provide yourself with opportunities to spot performance patterns and iron out weak points while building upon your strengths.

Your preparation training must be done with self-control. If you attempt to do long distances every day, at your intended marathon pace, you are likely to burn out and become exhausted within a few weeks. Instead, look to train six days a week, but for four of those training days run fairly manageable distances of 6.4–13km (4–8 miles) at an easy or mixed pace. For your fifth day, up the mileage and then, for the final training day of the week, do a significant distance at attempted race pace, building up from around 16km

Military Endurance

If the only option of getting somewhere is to walk or run, it is essential that military personnel can cope with covering long distances while carrrying their equipment. Elite soldiers may have to carry up to 40kg (88lb) of kit.

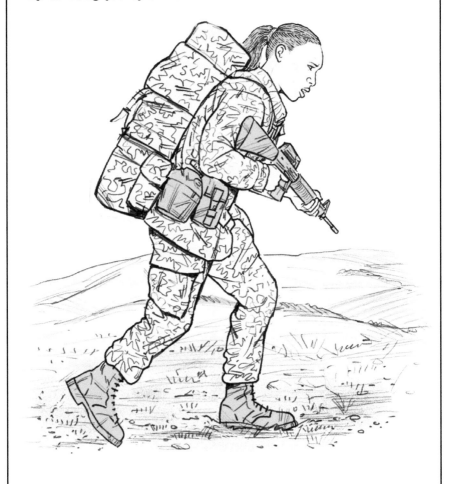

(10 miles) in week one and going up to around 32km (20 miles) in week 14. Weeks 15 and 16 should see you 'tapering' your training programme down in terms of distance run to prepare your body for the ordeal that lies ahead. During race week, have at least two rest days and only run two or three short distances at an easy pace. This way you will go into race day feeling fresh and energized.

Pacing Yourself

One sign of an inexperienced distance runner can be that he attacks every run at maximum pace, driving himself harder and harder despite his body loudly broadcasting various signals that it can't cope with the physical demands. Most experienced racers, by contrast, understand how to use a variety of pacing and speed in both their training runs and on race day.

Don't, for example, be afraid to walk certain parts of a run. Some associate the run/walk pattern as a beginner's technique, but in fact many ultra-distance runners necessarily incorporate walking as a deliberate part of their running strategy. Research, and empirical evidence from marathon athletes such as Jeff Galloway, suggests that periodically walking sections of a marathon can actually result in a significant improvement in times for intermediate runners. The walk periods give the body chance to

recuperate, preventing the runner 'hitting the wall' later on in the race, and producing faster running paces later on to compensate for the walked periods.

You can go into walk mode when your body dictates – if your breathing is becoming excessively laboured, or you feel your muscles weakening, drop into a brisk walk, get control of your breathing again, plus rehydrate with a good energy drink. After about a minute of walking, break into your run again and you should feel a distinct improvement in your energy levels. Alternatively, you can adopt a more regimented walk/run strategy. Many beginner and intermediate marathon runners have utilized a technique whereby they run 1.6km (1 mile) then walk for 60 seconds. Indeed, some marathon runners have produced sub 3:30 times using this very technique. Even if you don't want such a strict system, take note that walking for short periods during a race might not be to the detriment of your overall time.

In your training phase, a variety of running pace and technique will help you to achieve your best final race time. For straightforward distances, alternate runs between easy pace (at which you can hold a conversation), moderate pace (a sub-race pace at which you can speak a few words at a time) and race pace (you shouldn't be able to speak more than one or two words).

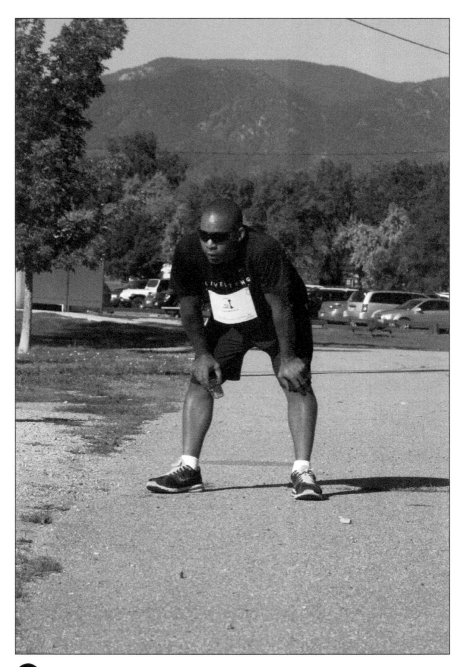

Opposite: It is important to increase runs at your own pace. If you feel you cannot speak more than a few words clearly, slow your pace or take a breather.

Mix things up by using interval training. Options include:

• **Increase/decrease** – start easy, but progressively turn up the speed until you are at race pace. Maintain this pace for a given period (1–5 minutes) then slacken the pace back down to easy again. Repeat this cycle several times during the duration of the run, making sure than you finish with at least 3km (2 miles) at an easy pace.

• **Interval runs** – interval running involves making switches in pace at regular, controlled periods or distances during your run. For example, after a 3.2km (2 mile) warm-up run, you could jog for 60 seconds then run at race-day pace for 60 seconds, so that your body becomes accustomed to applying sudden surges of power. The sprint sections will also raise your standard running pace if you practice this interval often enough. A distance-measured option (ideally suited to track running) would be to run at your best pace for 800m (2624ft) then drop back to a light jog for 400m (1312ft), repeating this cycle as many times as your training session allows.

• **Hill runs** – terrain as well as pace offers options for interval training. After warming up on the flat for a couple of miles, a section of steep incline will intensify effort, especially if you attempt to maintain the on-flat pace up the hill. You could also try running on different surfaces to alter pace and energy – a sandy beach is ideal for this.

• **Circuit runs** – here you build non-running exercises – such as star jumps, press-ups, squat thrusts or step-ups – into your running circuit, performing them at fixed points or at predetermined times. Circuit runs not only contribute to your all-over body fitness, they can also make your run more interesting, hence they are a good option if you feel your interest in running is waning. Just ensure that you catch your breath from the run before dropping down into the exercise; circuit runs are best performed in easy pace runs.

Interval training is a great way to increase your performance and keep your interest in your training programme. Military PTIs frequently use it as a way to build up fitness levels in their personnel, and the U.S. Army's *Physical Fitness Training* manual explains the technique and benefits: 'In interval training, a soldier exercises by running at a pace that is slightly faster than his race pace for short periods of time. This may be faster than the pace he wants to maintain during the next APFT [Army

Adductor Stretches

Adductor stretches before running can reduce the risk of leg or groin strain. They also improve the range of motion of the hips. Apply pressure evenly to the knees.

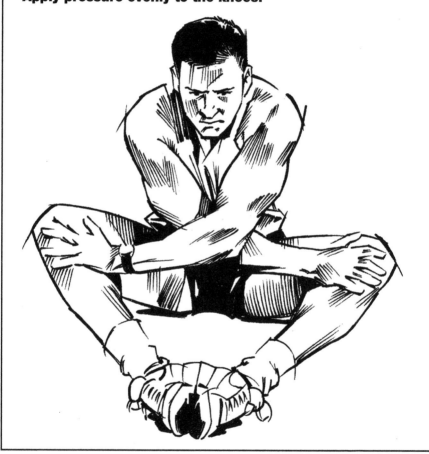

Physical Fitness Test] 2-mile run. He does this repeatedly with periods of recovery placed between periods of fast running. In this way, the energy systems used are allowed to recover, and the exerciser can do more fast-paced running in a given workout than if he ran continuously without

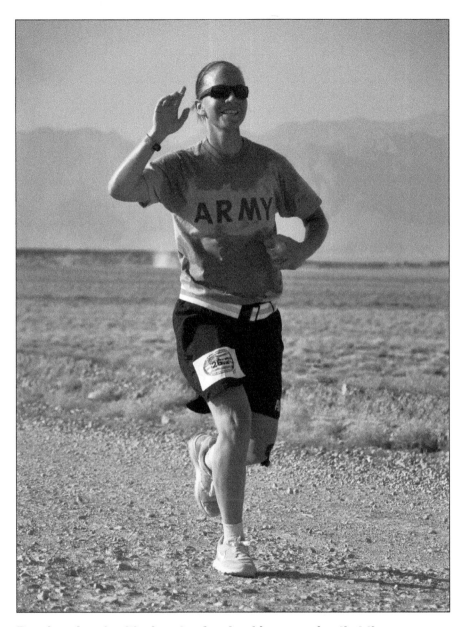

Running gives healthy boosts of endorphins, meaning that the more you exercise, the better you will feel, both physically and mentally.

Race Preparation Tips

- If possible, try to see the racecourse before race day. Cycling around it is a convenient option, stopping regularly to make notes about course features in a notebook. You could also run certain sections of the course in advance.
- Control your diet. Start carb-loading four days before the race, and fluid-loading two days before. The night before the race eat a carb-rich meal of about 1000 calories, and on race day an 800-calorie meal two hours before the race will give you plenty of energy.
- Cut your toenails.
- If you are staying in a hotel the night before the race, taking your own pillow helps ensure a decent night's sleep.
- Write down all the race information as simple notes so that you aren't wading through lots of paperwork to get to essential race information.
- Make sure that any shoes or clothing you are using for the race day has been 'broken in' well in advance of the actual race.
- Time your training runs for the same time of day as the race run. This way your body will be familiar with exertion at the right time of day.

resting. This type of intermittent training can also be used with activities such as cycling, swimming, bicycling, rowing and road marching' (2-3).

Group Training

If you are going to do any sort of competitive racing, or if your times have hit a plateau and you are looking to push yourself further, your best option might be to utilize what the U.S. military calls 'Ability Group Running' (AGR). Field Manual 21-20 again explains the core principles involved: 'AGR lets soldiers train in groups of near-equal ability.

Each group runs at a pace intense enough to produce a training effect for that group and each soldier in it. Leaders should program these runs for specific lengths of time, not miles

Standing Quad Stretch

You should feel a quadriceps stretch along the front of your leg. Keep the knee of the supporting leg soft and use a wall or chair for balance.

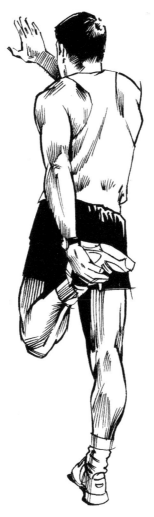

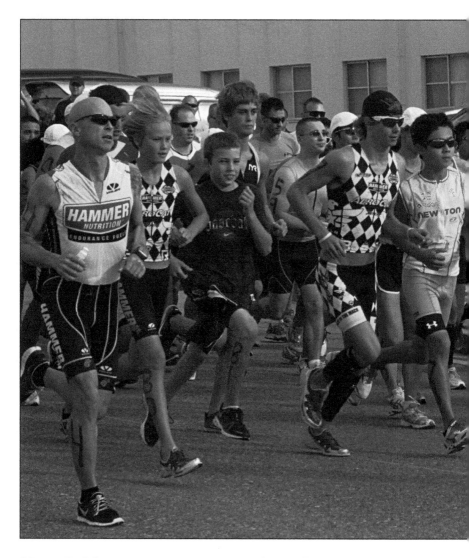

Above: Training runs or ability group running are good ways of training with supportive, like-minded people, as well as challenging yourself against others.

to be run. This procedure lets more-fit groups run a greater distance than the less-fit groups in the same time period, thus enabling every soldier to improve' (2-3).

As running is such a popular

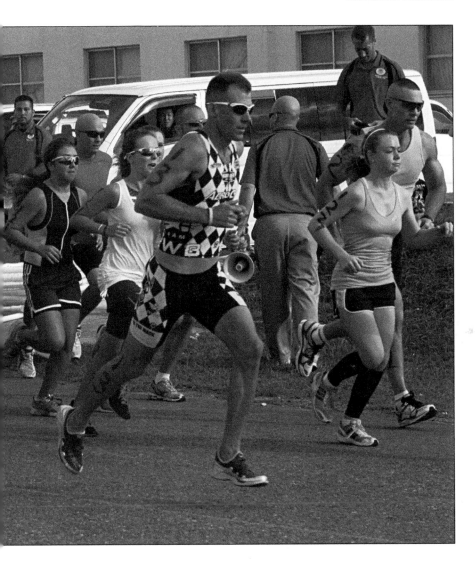

sport, most regions will have clubs taking on new members. AGR is most productive when the group is of near-equal ability – natural competitive effect will ensure that the group as an entity pushes itself hard, with a cumulative improvement in running times. It is important in any group run, however, to set out the aims and ground rules clearly. A run leader should define the type of run, its route and policies on practices such

Quad Lifts

Quad lifts strengthen the muscles around the front of the knees, giving the joint greater stability for running. This lift can be a good exercise when building up strength following knee injuries.

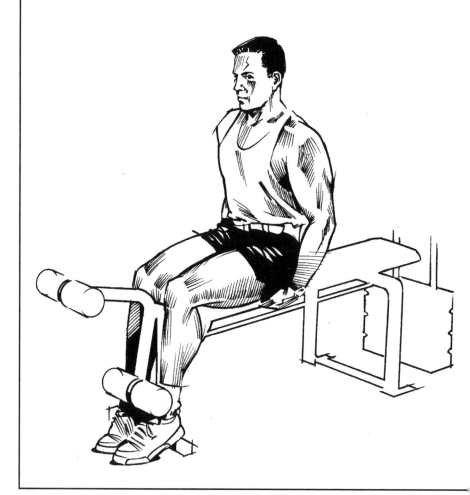

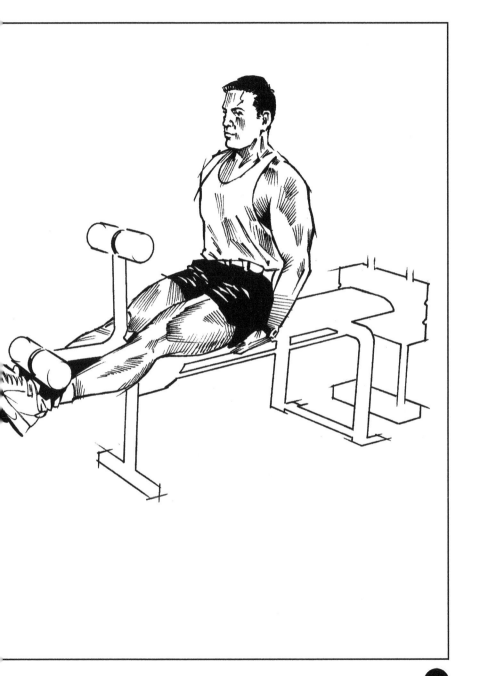

U.S. Army Tip – Fartlek Training

In Fartlek training, another type of CR training sometimes called speed play, the soldier varies the intensity (speed) of the running during the workout. Instead of running at a constant speed, he starts with very slow jogging. When ready, he runs hard for a few minutes until he feels the need to slow down. At this time he recovers by jogging at an easy pace. This process of alternating fast and recovery running (both of varying distances) gives the same results as interval training. However, neither the running nor recovery interval is timed, and the running is not done on a track. For these reasons, many runners prefer Fartlek training to interval training.

– U.S. Army, FM 21-20, 2-6

as walking sections. Above all, make sure that you are comfortable within the group's personalities, and in a relaxed state of mind. Most groups are enthusiastic and welcoming, so will likely add to your social life as well as your running times.

Race Day

A race day is the culmination of all your training. In the immediate minutes before the race, warm up and stretch out *gently* – don't do anything too vigorous prior to the start. By taking your place alongside ranks of other runners, you are guaranteed an extra burst of adrenaline and motivation. This is good, but there are dangers. Chief among them is

that you set off at a pace you simply cannot maintain for the duration of the race. Instead, establish a brisk but comfortable pace – ideally about 10–15 seconds slower than your ideal race pace – and don't allow yourself to be pushed on quicker by others passing you; if you maintain your pace you will pass many of them later on in the race. Stay relaxed and loose. By conserving your energy, you give yourself the capacity for turning up the pace significantly in the last 10km (6.2 miles) of the race, which is where you can hit your optimum pace.

'Hitting the wall' is a common, sometimes insurmountable, challenge for marathon runners. It is literally caused by the muscles running out of glucose to supply their energy needs. The symptoms are sapping: limbs feel like unwieldy lumps of lead and every step is mentally and physically exhausting. Prevention is obviously better than cure. Keep very well hydrated during the race, taking on hydration fluids every 20 minutes. Also refuel with carb-rich snacks every hour. Combine these good practices with proper pacing and you stand a good chance of avoiding hitting the wall in the last stages of the race. If you do, mental tenacity is the thing that will get you through.

Remember that marathons are as much about psychology as stamina. One trick to help you cope with the distance is to break the race down into multiple small sections, and see each section as a separate event that you can complete comfortably. Perhaps tie each section with different styles of music through your headphones. The music for the first 10km (6 miles) could, say, be pacey but relaxed, while during the last 10km (6 miles) of the race the music could be more aggressive in rhythm and character. Basically, draw on any mental technique you can to keep one leg moving in front of the other.

Off-road Endurance

City marathons are the most popular long-distance running events, attended by tens of thousands of people worldwide every year. At the beginning of this chapter, however, we listed some wilderness ultra-marathons that are only attempted by the most committed of athletes. Make no mistake – running more than 160km (100 miles) in a few days requires serious preparation and training, with weekly distances of up to and beyond 80km (50 miles). More than that, you also need to cope with difficult terrain and climate in the most direct way.

We start with the most basic form of off-road running – hill running. Hill running is a superb route to endurance and muscular strength, and has the ancillary benefit of making running on the flat seem that much easier. Hills and mountains come in all shapes and sizes, and the races available to hill runners vary from relatively sedate ambling routes through to terrifying Alpine races that blur the lines between climbing and running.

Naturally you should take a graduated approach to hill training, working your way up from basic hills of around a ten per cent incline to more challenging gradients and distances. In military training, for example, tough tests such as the UK Special Forces 'Long Drag' are introduced after the recruits have already had several weeks of slogging up peaks, thereby building up the essential lower-limb strength and respiratory stamina.

The key to successful hill running is building up endurance. These recruits need to avoid using energy-sapping movements and keep their pace consistent.

In terms of basic hill-running technique, your primary goal is to build up rhythmic pace and breathing, despite the irregular terrain. Keep your arms loose and your head and neck upright; drop your eyes and not your head if you need to check out the close terrain. As the incline steepens, shorten your step but try to keep the same pace of turnover you were maintaining on the flat. Push lightly off the surface of the hill and avoid making large sprinting strides if possible, as these sap energy. (You can, of course, build fast intervals into your hill running as a specific training technique, if you choose.)

Plot your route carefully up the slope if a well-worn track is not easily visible. Avoid sections of loose earth or shingle, or very thick grasses, which can hide ankle-snapping potholes. An obvious goal for your run is the summit, but aim to run a little beyond to allow your body to adjust to the stop – don't just stop dead at the top, as this runs the risk of lactic acid-induced cramps.

Downhill running presents challenges all of its own. The temptation is to give in to gravity and allow speed to build up. Not only does this have a risk of your run

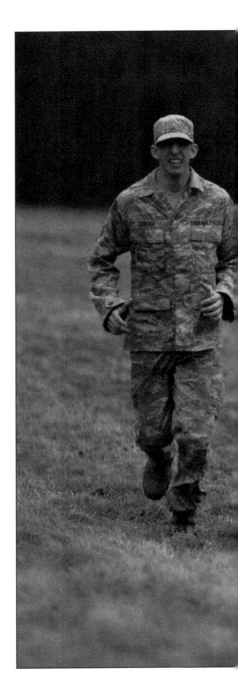

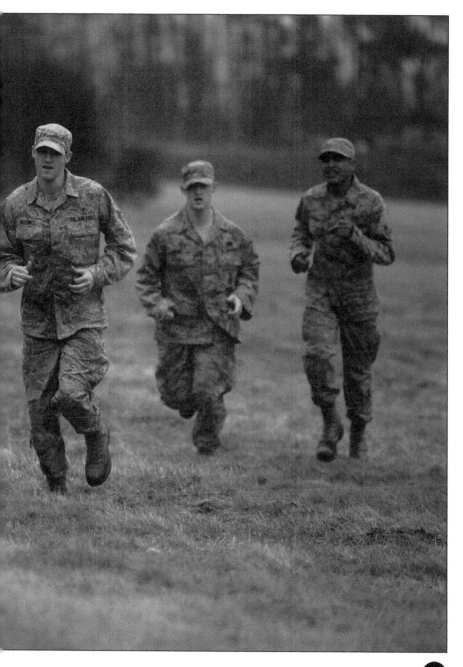

Royal Marine Advanced Combat Fitness Test – Endurance Marches

Day 1 is a 20km (12.4 mile) endurance march over varied terrain, which at least 6km (3.7 miles) is to be off metalled roads and is to be completed in a max time of 3 hr 30 min, but not less than 3 hr 25 min, carrying a total load of 31.30kgs (69lbs) consisting of PLCE, bergen and personal wpn. The time allowed is inclusive of any time taken for rehydration stops, safety checks or any other essential administrative activity, which is deemed necessary by the Conducting Officer.

Day 2 comprises of two parts, they are:

Part 1 – Consists of a 20km (12 mile) endurance march, over varied terrain, which at least 6km (3.7 miles) to be off metalled roads, and is to be completed in a maximum time of 3 hr, but not less that 2 hr 55 min, carrying a load of 25kg (55lb). The time allowed is inclusive of any time taken for re-hydration stops, safety checks or any other essential administrative activity which is deemed necessary by the Conducting Officer.

Part 2 – On completion of Part 1 all personnel are to complete a range of RMT selected by the Comd, in consultation with Unit PTI. These are to be a minimum of 3 tasks, from those listed in Table 8 on page 30, which best represent role-related operational requirements for anaerobic muscular endurance (speed), muscular strength and combat agility, each individual RMT is only to be used once per test.

– *Royal Marine Fitness Tests,* p.59

becoming uncontrollable, terminating in a fall, but the chances of sprained ankle or knee go up commensurately. Instead, keep your body upright to the horizontal, and don't bounce off the face of the inclines – keep your feet close to the surface of the incline and don't land them with heavy impact. If you feel that your running speed is getting away from you, shorten the length of stride until you are back in control of your speed.

Special Terrains

Ultra-marathons, like Special Forces training, often take the runner into special terrains and climates that add extra challenges to the completion of the fitness challenge. Desert, jungle, mountain, snowscape – all can be deadly to runners and soldiers who don't possess survival awareness and the right kit.

It is impossible in this limited space to provide a complete guide to wilderness survival in all different and possibly hostile terrains. Needless to say, if you are undertaking an ultra-marathon in a wilderness setting, do your survival research and relevant training well in advance. Race organizers will usually be more than happy to advise you on the special physical requirements of the race, and online race forums are also a treasure trove of practical information provided by those who have already completed such challenges.

Here, however, we will look at a few core considerations for racing in extreme environments, incorporating some of the hard-acquired advice given by the military community whose job it is to conduct operations in all manner of wilderness.

Desert

For desert runs, the obvious threat to manage is that from the unforgiving sun, which presents dangers in the form of sunburn, heat exhaustion and heat stroke. The heat of the sun is compounded by heat gain, which refers to the heat reflected from sand and rocks, and held in heated wind-blown sand.

Other perils of the desert include sandstorms that can reduce visibility to practically zero, heat mirages and shimmer, which hamper the accurate navigation so crucial in a largely featureless environment, and some perfectly nasty biting creatures, such as highly venomous snakes, scorpions and spiders.

The advice given by the U.S. Army's *Survival* manual about conducting operations in desert regions is solid and practical:

- *Make sure you tell someone where you are going and when you will return.*
- *Watch for signs of heat injury. If someone complains of tiredness or wanders away from the group, he may be a heat casualty.*
- *Drink water at least once an hour.*
- *Get in the shade when resting; do not lie directly on the ground.*
- *Do not take off your shirt and work during the day.*
- *Check the colour of your urine. A light colour means you are drinking enough water,*

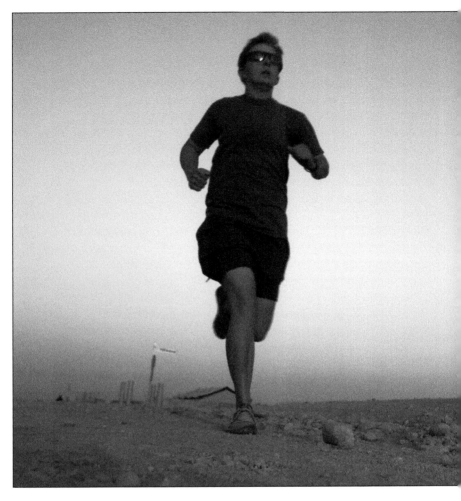

a dark colour means you need to drink more.
– FM 3-05-70, *Survival, 13-12*

The first two points emphasize group or paired running. Even in a race, make sure that you can see others, either racers or race organizers, and unless you are an expert navigator and survivalist, don't head off on your own into a scorching wilderness. The points about shade and rehydration should be followed religiously. Races such as the Marathon des Sables and the Death Valley run push against what would be good survival advice by conducting heavy exertion at the

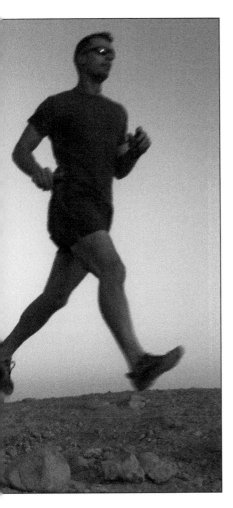

Left: Keeping yourself hydrated is vital during desert runs. Set regular hydration stops, typically every 20–30 minutes.

will increase your sweating through exertion.) Aim to consume about 2500–3000 calories a day.

Your clothing is also critical for desert runs. The military advice is to keep your full uniform on, as exposing bare skin to extreme heat leaves you more open to heat stroke and sunburn. Wear UV-protective leggings and running top, plus a running cap with full neck protection. Apply factor 50 sun cream to any exposed skin, refreshing the coverage at one-hour intervals.

A big problem in desert running is that of sand filling up your footware, introducing an abrasive substance that quickly produces painful blisters and foot infections. Purpose-designed desert gaiters, which are fitted around the ankle and over the top of the shoe, will help to prevent this problem to an extent, although extremely fine sand dust will still find its way in and should be emptied from the shoe regularly. Many runners fashion their own gaiters from sections of non-porous parachute-type fabric, gluing the bottom edge of the fabric to the rim of the shoe and tying the body of the fabric to the leg just above the knee.

Desert running is extremely hard on legs and feet. A decent antiseptic

very hottest parts of the day. Drink a good rehydration fluid containing electrolytes every 20–30 minutes, and for nutrition rely upon energy bars and light energy meals – nuts, dried fruit and basic porridges are good. Avoid any which are heavy in fats. (Any foodstuffs should also be as light as possible to carry, as additional weight

ointment is an essential part of your running kit for treating blisters and minor cuts, which can get infected quickly in a desert climate. You can also tape your feet with a self-adhesive tape such as Mefix, concentrating on the parts of the feet where blisters are likely to occur. Most desert runners also carry a pair of lightweight collapsible walking poles, which are a practical means of both reducing the pressure on the legs and also of retaining stability and speed (about a 30 per cent improvement) when running over soft, sandy surfaces.

When running in the desert, don't forget good sports sunglasses. Advanced types include insert sections so you can affix prescription lenses of various types (sunglasses and clear) as required, and go for a design that wraps around the eyes to protect you from glare from the ground as much as direct sunlight from above.

Jungle

Jungle is arguably the most demanding terrain for the ultra-runner, hence only an elite few venture into this wilderness. Jungle terrain is extremely variable, ranging from towering tropical rainforests down to foot-sucking swamps. Yet all have elements in common – heat, very high humidity, an over-abundance of dangerous wildlife and tortuous, ankle-snapping terrain.

Running through the jungle is complicated by incessant obstacles, plus the problems of navigation when the only thing you can see is vegetation all around. You should be properly versed in jungle navigation techniques before you even consider a jungle ultra-marathon, and don't think you can just rely on a GPS system. The U.S. Army *Survival* manual gives advice to its soldiers, applicable to runners, about how to 'see' through the jungle foliage:

> To move easily, you must develop 'jungle eye,' that is, you should not concentrate on the pattern of bushes and trees to your immediate front. You must focus on the jungle further out and find natural breaks in the foliage. Look through the jungle, not at it. Stop and stoop down occasionally to look along the jungle floor. This action may reveal game trails that you can follow.

– FM 3-05-70, *Survival*, 14-6

When running in a jungle environment, place your feet consciously and carefully, and don't go faster than the terrain allows. Twist around dense foliage rather than attempting to bludgeon your way through, although the occasional swing of a machete may be necessary depending on the type

Marathon de Sable Gear

Temperates in the Sahara can exceed the mid-fifties centigrade. This runner is wearing appropriate gear, including sunglasses, neck shield and sand boots.

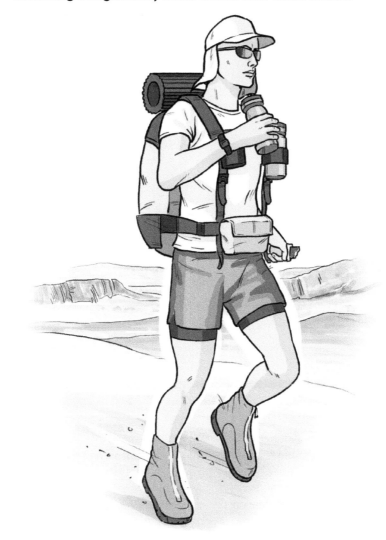

Fell-running Terrain

When fell running, choose your route before you set off, avoiding unstable surfaces, excessive inclines and precipitous drops.

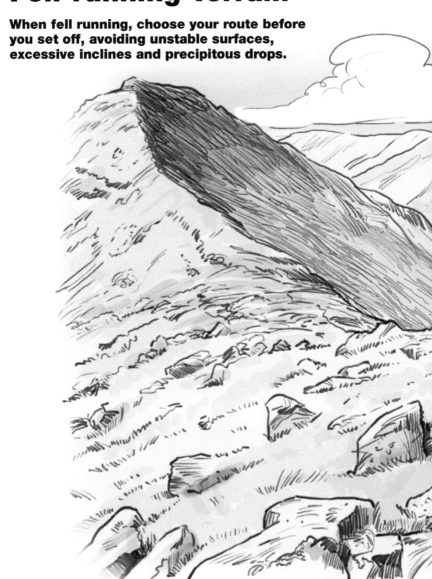

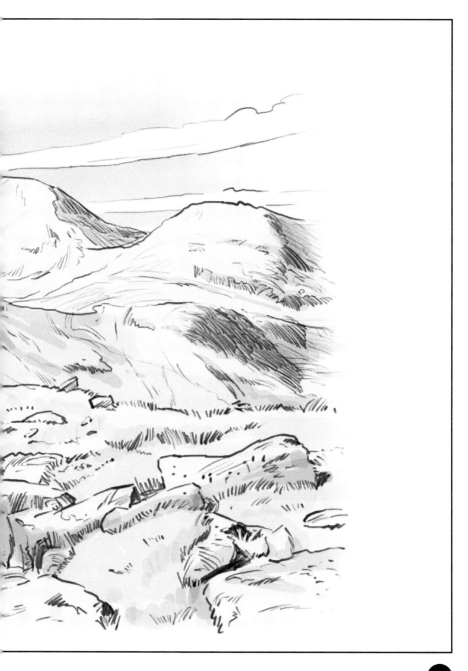

of course. Make up your speed when you reach stretches of good track, often alongside rivers. Avoid reaching out and grabbing foliage with your hands to stabilize yourself; many jungle plants bear thorns, some with poisonous content. For this reason, wearing a good strong pair of jungle gloves is recommended. When you stop for a rest, look carefully at your surroundings. Snakes, spiders and other creatures often like to shelter under pieces of wood or under rocks, so before sitting down on a log or similar feature, check beneath it with a long stick. If you do encounter or flush out a dangerous animal, move away from it slowly and carefully.

The greatest problem in a jungle is humidity, and occasional heavy rain. In the jungle everything is soaking wet pretty much all the time, and it is almost impossible to dry out clothing in these conditions. Keep anything that needs to stay dry – spare clothing, socks, electric equipment, maps, etc. – wrapped up in double layers of plastic in your pack. The pack itself should be close fitting with no loose straps or flapping drinking tubes; anything that sticks out from your body will get caught on foliage. Your pack should include plenty of artificial illumination for night stages, including head torch and light sticks.

The humidity can be particularly sapping for those who aren't used to it. Ideally, spend a week or two in the host climate before the race, conducting some shorter distance runs and getting your body used to the demands about to be placed upon it. Such advice applies to all extreme environment runs.

Mountains

In the section on hill running above, we have already explained some of the basic techniques for running around precipitous environments. Some ultra-marathons take the sport to a whole new level (literally) by racing at high altitudes. The Beyond the Ultimate Mountain Ultra, for example, reaches altitudes of more than 2743m (9000ft), where the air is thin and runners face the perils of altitude sickness. The higher you go, the less oxygen is available to fuel your efforts, hence high-altitude runners have to put in maximum effort at every stage of the race.

Acclimatization is the best way to ensure that you run efficiently at high altitude. Ideally, aim to move into the race altitude zone two weeks before the start of the event to give your respiratory system and your muscles time to adjust to the conditions. For many international runners, who have other lives apart from race days, such a prolonged vacation is rarely an option. In these cases, it is ironically best to arrive at the race location just before the start, beginning the race with the energy levels of the lower

Tips for Running in Snow

- Wear either studded trail shoes or fit your regular running shoes with ice grips. Carry a spare pair of grips in your backpack.
- Ensure that your running shoes have waterproof uppers, such as Gore-Tex.
- Wear thick woollen socks and gloves, and ensure that your ears are also covered by a woollen hat. Frostbite can attack the extremities in minutes, and by running you are increasing the windchill factor.
- Ideally run on compacted areas of snow. Take small steps as you run on fresh snow, and always be on the lookout for patches of ice.
- Wear a waterproof outer layer with a thermal layer beneath.
- Plan your route carefully. Avoid stopping at any time, as your sweat will start to freeze very quickly and your body temperature will drop precipitously.

altitudes and (hopefully) adjusting to the conditions as you go along. Should you at any point start to experience symptoms of altitude sickness – trouble breathing, severe headaches, nausea, disturbed vision, lapses in consciousness – then stop racing and immediately get to lower altitudes, under medical supervision.

Training for mountain racing involves focusing your attention on effort rather than pace. Increase the intensity of your training sessions so that you are working at high heart and breathing rates. By doing this at sea level, at least, you will improve your VO_2 max (the maximum capacity of a person's body to transport and use oxygen), which will support you during the high-altitude runs. When running in mountains, also implement a diligent rehydration routine – some high-altitude regions can be as dry as deserts, and dehydration can be a serious problem, especially as cold weather tricks the mind into thinking the body doesn't need fluids.

Running in extreme terrains is precarious but rewarding. Those who have tackled ultra-marathons often report not only a sense of athletic achievement, but also a spiritual reconnection with the landscape through which they have travelled.

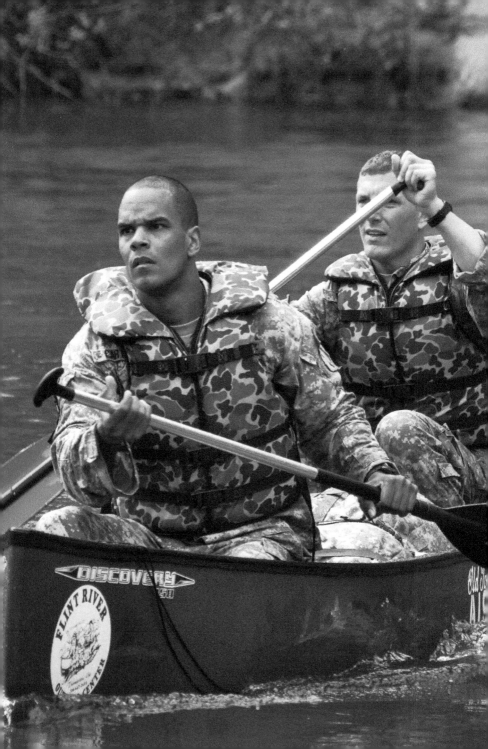

It is not a coincidence that some of the world's most elite units are those that have a specialism in aquatic warfare. Being air-breathing mammals, humans are undeniably intended for land-based existence. Hence those who chose to master the world of water are essentially fighting against an alien environment. The seas and oceans are replete with threats that can, and do, claim thousands of lives every year. Drowning is obviously the chief danger, exacerbated by factors such as strong currents and hypothermia. Powerful waves can destroy large ships, never mind vulnerable human swimmers. The Earth's waters are also host to a submerged world of dangerous creatures, from venomous jellyfish to massive, predatory species of shark. Soldiers such as those of the U.S. Navy SEALs and the British Special Boat Service (SBS) are, therefore, men of unique physical and mental makeup.

In this chapter we will look at aquatic extreme fitness challenges, focusing principally on the activities of distance swimming and rowing, with a look at relatively recent extreme sports such as free-diving. The seas and oceans in particular are uniquely dangerous places, and even experienced athletes can go

• •

Opposite: Military aquatic training focus on combat swimming and small-boat handling.

4

Some 70 per cent of the world's surface is covered by water. This means that extreme aquatic challenges are readily available for those who want to test themselves to the limit.

Extreme Water

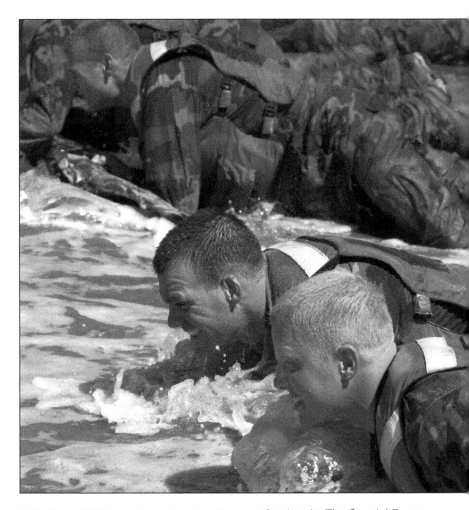

U.S. Navy SEALs undertake a 'surf torture' exercise, building levels of mental endurance.

from normality to crisis in minutes if they are caught unawares. Therefore, those who intend to pursue aquatic challenges are urged to take proper training alongside experienced professionals. The Special Forces invest thousands of dollars in training their operatives to survive in water environments, so never believe you can take short cuts with safety.

Body Effects

The U.S. Navy SEALs are the most famous of the aquatic Special Forces,

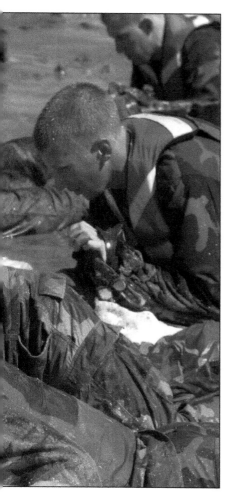

might also have to carry weapons and other equipment during the arm-breaking transit.

SEAL training introduces the recruits to the full spectrum of dangers posed by the seas. First, the sea is a swirling mass of energy, directing that energy into currents and waves. The currents can take even the strongest swimmer away from his intended destination, especially in the form of riptides. Accounting for a total of 80 per cent of causes for lifeguard rescues, riptides are essentially strong backflows of water from the shoreline, the current breaking through the waves and pushing out into open water. Those caught in riptides suddenly find themselves carried out to sea at speed. Waves add their own set of dangers. Not only do they have an impact on the directional progress of a swimmer, powerful shorebreak waves can either smash directly onto the swimmer or hurl him against shoreline rocks, both inflicting serious impact injuries.

Aquatic environments also present a challenge for the baseline functions of the human physiology. The most serious consideration is the effect of water temperature on body temperature. Experienced swimmers have long noted the apparent paradox that a certain temperature on land feels much colder in the water. The primary reason for this is water's excellent qualities of conduction – its ability to transfer heat. Water presses

or at least the one about which we have decent training information. The SEALs are trained in the arts of amphibious combat and survival by any means, including the simple expedient of swimming long distances to shore from a deployment vessel. Not only do they need to be able to do this in full swimming kit, but they

Canoe Race

Canoe racing can take the form of a marathon, sprint or slalom. The longest canoe marathon takes place on the Yukon and covers 1600km (1000 miles) of the river.

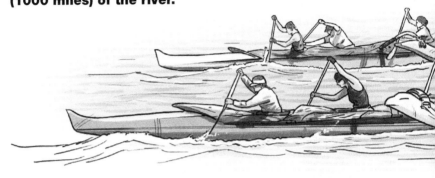

directly against any submerged skin, and therefore rapidly draws out heat from the body. Elementary physics tells us that two objects of heat contrast, in contact with one another, and will transfer heat to the point that both reach a common temperature. The sea, however, is such a huge mass that it will simply continue to chill the person until, if the water is cold enough, the swimmer goes into hypothermia. The problem is made worse when swimming by convection: as the swimmer's body warms water, the warm water rises and is replaced by cold water from below. This cycle continues, so cold water is constantly playing across the surface of the skin, accelerating heat loss.

Buoyancy

The physical properties of water have other effects on the body. One is the influence of buoyancy. Water exhibits an upward force that creates the weightless sensation experienced by swimmers (salt content also makes sea water more buoyant than fresh water). A human adds to the buoyancy by virtue of certain body parts, especially their air-filled lungs – the centre of buoyancy in people is

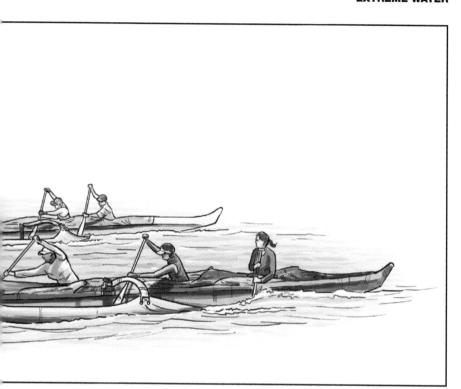

the middle of the chest, just beneath the solar plexus. The U.S. Navy's *Navy Swimming and Water Survival Manual* clarifies that 'Water has a specific gravity of 1. The specific gravity of other objects is compared to this number. Objects with a specific gravity of less than 1 float, while objects with a specific gravity greater than 1 sink. Specific gravity among humans varies by muscle mass, amount of fat and bone density. Some individuals will not float, even with a full breath of air, while executing a survival float' (3.4). The last point is important for the survival considerations that take precedence in all extreme swimming. Don't think that you can rely on floating alone as a survival measure, but like a U.S. Navy SEAL you will have to perfect your own techniques of 'drown-proofing'.

Distance Swimming

As with running, the sport of swimming has also recently created a whole new series of endurance events. For many years, at least in Europe, the major goal of distance swimmers was to cross the frigid 33.1km (20.6 miles) of the Straits of Dover between France and England.

Bog Snorkelling

Although a snorkel and flippers are worn, traditional swimming strokes should not – usually can not – be used when bog snorkelling, meaning that ever more inventive methods are used.

The first man to make an unassisted swim of the Channel was the stalwart Captain Matthew Webb, who made the crossing on 24–25 August 1875 in 21 hours 45 minutes. Since that inaugural event, more than 700 people have made the crossing. In 2010, quadruple amputee Philippe Croizon also swam the Channel, propelling himself via fins attached to his prosthetic limbs. Croizon perfectly embodies the spirit of those who take on extreme fitness challenges, refusing to accept limitations placed upon them by the physical world. Alongside him rank individuals such as the Australian–British swimmer Penny Palfrey, who swam unassisted (no swimming cage to protect from sharks, no wet suit) 112km (70 miles)

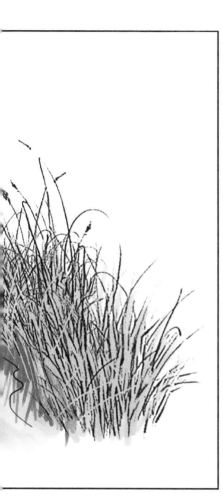

of Swimming), recognized by the International Olympic Committee (IOC), classifies swims of or greater than 10km (6 miles) in open water as aquatic marathons, and there are literally dozens of these events conducted around the world, either in inland waters or open seas. Some of the most challenging ultra-swimming marathons, apart from the English Channel, include the Catalina Channel between Santa Catalina Island and southern California at 32.5km (20.2 miles) and the dangerous waters of the Cook Strait between the North and South Islands of New Zealand – a distance of 22km (14 miles). Furthermore, long-distance swimming is an integral part of triathlon events.

Swimming in Open Sea

Although many people conduct distance-swimming challenges in swimming pools, the majority of them take place in the open sea. For those used to the calm and controlled conditions of a pool, the transition to open-water swimming can be a shock. Currents, waves, cold temperatures, aquatic wildlife (some of it dangerous) and the disorientation of a featureless sea are all traps for the unprepared. Much U.S. Navy SEAL Second Phase training is focused on making the candidates at home in the open-water environment. The horrible near-hypothermic ordeals in the surf are designed to train the candidate to both recognize the

between Grand Cayman and Little Cayman islands in the Caribbean in 2012, setting a new world record for distance swimming.

The Channel crossing is just one of literally hundreds of distance swims open to those with exceptional fitness and a dogged spirit. Fédération Internationale de Natation (International Federation

Rebreather Outfit

Used for scuba diving, a rebreather suit has a device for absorbing the carbon dioxide expelled in breath, literally enabling the wearer to rebreathe or re-use the same air.

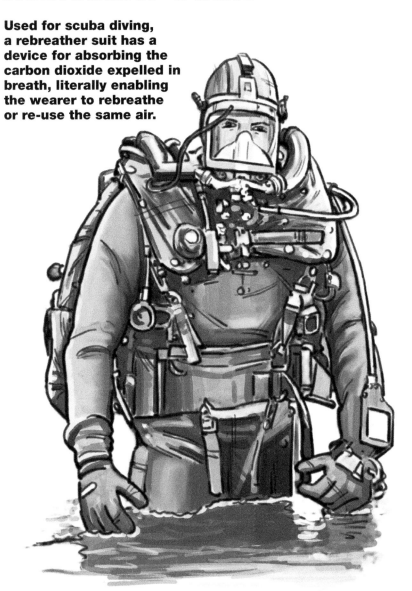

Life Jacket

Invest in a high-quality life jacket, featuring safety kit such as a water-activated light, whistle and even GPS locator.

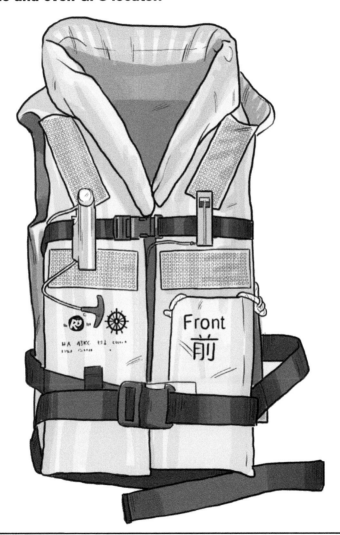

Escaping a Rip Tide

Here the swimmer escapes the rip tide by swimming across and through the current, rather than attempting to swim directly against the current.

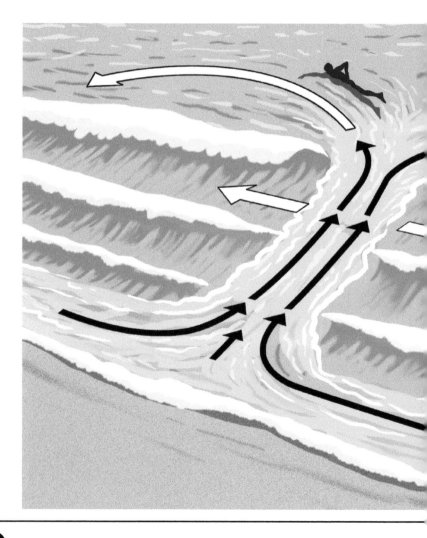

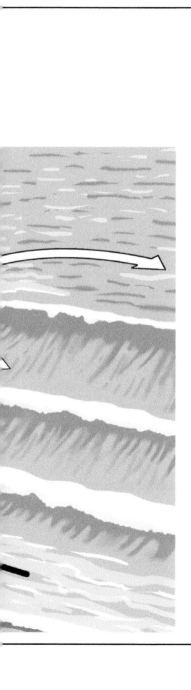

Escaping a Riptide

As part of basic training, combat swimmers are taught the fundamental principles of how to escape riptides:

- Try to gain a footing on the floor if possible, as standing on the seabed will usually enable you to resist the pull of the riptide.
- Don't panic. The riptide will only take you out, not under, so if you start to struggle simply relax and float on your back for a while to regain your energy.
- Swim parallel to the shoreline to escape the riptide. Riptides are generally quite narrow, typically being around 30–45m (98–148ft) wide, so by swimming across the riptide you will eventually break out the side of the current. Then swim to shore, avoiding the line of the riptide.
- If you can't do this, note that most riptides will disperse about 100m (328ft) from the shoreline. Then choose a safe point further along the beach and swim to it.

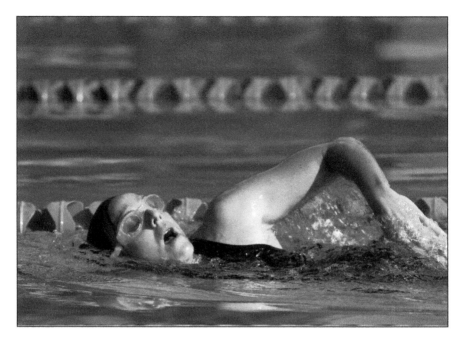

Long-distance lane swimming is an excellent way to build all-over tone, stamina and lung capacity.

symptoms of hypothermia, and also to see whether the candidate can control mental functions even when very cold. Distance swims of several miles are conducted in a variety of water conditions, from coastal to open blue sea. During these swims, the candidate will have to perform a variety of military tasks, including life saving, reconnaissance and demolitions diving. The intensity of the swims is also varied, from easy swims of around 1.6km (1 mile) – albeit conducted after the candidate has just run about 10km (6 miles) – to high-intensity 0.4km (0.25-mile) sprint swims, again interspersed with land-based activities.

Ultra-swimming marathons are rarely parts of military amphibious programmes (as far as the author is aware), principally because a soldier would never use such distances as part of a deployment strategy. Yet as we shall see in this chapter, the training methods of units such as the SEALs have some direct applications to extreme swimming challenges.

Preparation
To even consider attempting an ultra swim you should naturally be a good and durable swimmer in the first place. At a minimum, you should be

U.S. Navy Tip – Panic and Acclimatization

People must be capable of thinking rationally in the water before they can be safe or learn new water skills. Thinking rationally requires adjustment to the differences between the land and the water. Different physical properties of water cause changes in the human body that inexperienced swimmers must learn to cope with before becoming acclimated, comfortable and safe. Changes on the human body produced by the water include sudden temperature change, wetness, pressure increase and the feeling of weightlessness. The weight of water makes breathing more difficult due to water pressure acting on the chest. Adjusting to these changes can cause increased metabolic and anxiety rates as students 'tense up'. Increased metabolic and anxiety rates caused by tensing up are often the cause of fear and panic. Repeated exposure and practice of Mental and Physical Adjustment to the Water skills in a controlled, comfortable environment allows students to overcome fear by repeated exposure and acclimatization to the differences between the water environment and the land environment.

– U.S. Navy, *Naval Swimmer and Instructor's Manual*, 8.5

able to maintain 3km/h (2mph) for many hours – the Channel crossing, for example, takes around 12–16 hours – but professional distance swimmers can achieve speeds of more than double that pace.

Preparation for an ultra-swimming event requires that you find a safe and accessible stretch of open water in which you can conduct regular practice swims. This can be more difficult than it sounds, as an ideal swimming ground might be within a busy shipping lane, and swimming there could result in your being arrested by the local coastguard. Always consult the coastguard authorities about places where you will be permitted to swim, or, better still, join a local distance-swimming

Front Crawl

An effective front crawl depends upon several key elements: a) the neck and body should be in good alignment; b) the breathing is coordinated with the strokes; and c) the arms make a smooth slicing motion through the water.

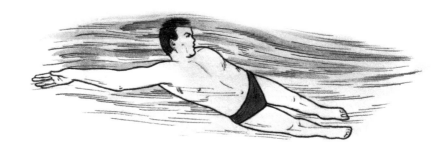

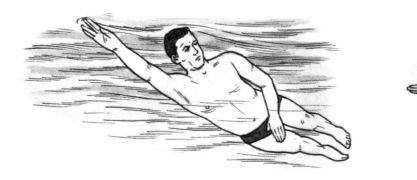

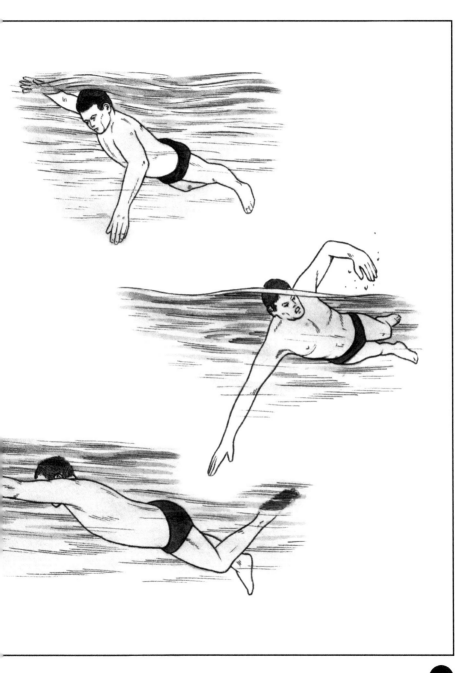

White-water Rafting

Rivers are graded for their difficulty in rafting, from Grade 1 (basic) to 6 (extreme skill). Grade 6 is considered so dangerous that injury or even death are likely, not rare.

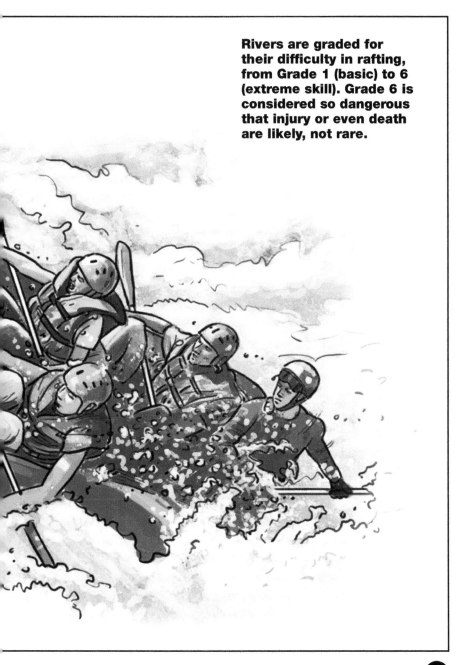

Passing Water – Long-distance Swimming

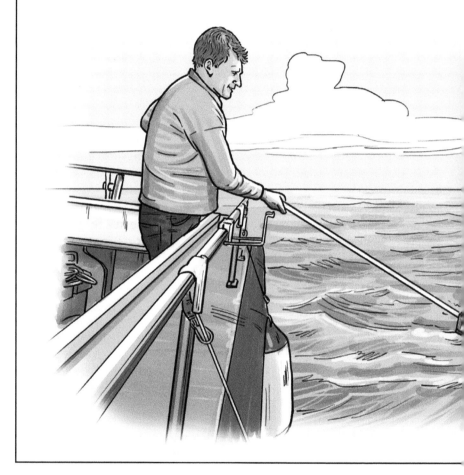

group who are already well-informed about the swimming regulations. One legal consideration – if you are swimming between different countries, ensure that you inform the authorities on both sides, otherwise you might be treated as an illegal immigrant when you

is important information. The sea's currents, tide and state will prevent you from swimming in a direct line from point A to point B.

Indeed many ultra swims actually describe an S or Z shape over the duration, requiring a start point that allows for these directional variations. The final shape of course partly relies on the speed and strength of your swimming stroke.

Support Team

Anyone attempting an ultra swim will usually be accompanied by a support person/team in a kayak or small boat. The support team will give navigational guidance throughout the swim, as at water level in a featureless sea maintaining a true bearing by sight alone is almost impossible. The support team will also provide food and drink throughout the swim; this is passed to the swimmer via a pole or by hand, or by the items being placed in floating containers, in turn attached to a rope (at least 15m/50ft in length to allow for boat drift) and thrown into the path of the swimmer. (For some distance events, the swimmer may actually board a vessel to consume food and drink, re-entering the water afterwards to continue the race.) Energy gel packs and other foodstuffs can be tied to the side of water bottles with thick elastic bands, and the addition of a chemical light stick will make the items much easier to find in low-light conditions or at night. If

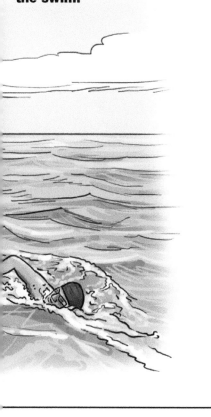

Dehydration can be as serious a problem in long-distance swimming as in long-distance running. Your support team should pass you water of measured quantities at timed intervals throughout the swim.

triumphantly reach your destination. The coastguard is also a useful source of information about sea conditions along your intended swim route. This

Snorkeling Gear

A mask, snorkel and fins are all that is required for snorkeling. Split fins are thought to improve the swimmer's speed through their propeller-like effect.

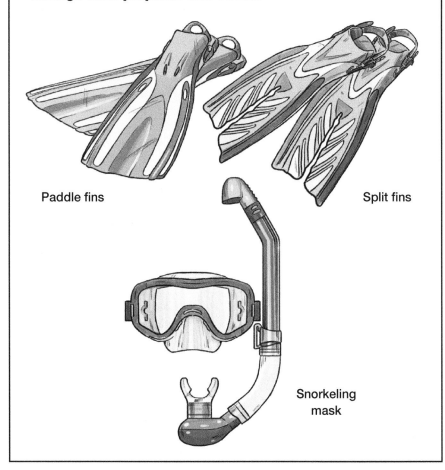

Paddle fins

Split fins

Snorkeling
mask

you are swimming against a time, you will need to keep your feeds as short as possible – ideally under a minute or even under 30 seconds. Feeding typically takes place on the hour, increasing to on the half hour as the race goes on and your energy levels start to flag. The swimmer should always ensure that his or her support team are experienced in helping people through ultra-marathons; any inefficiencies on their part could result in either a failed challenge at best, or a life-threatening emergency at worst.

Hazards

Even supposedly warm seas are often capable of inducing hypothermia if an individual is submerged long enough without artificially raising his body temperature. The end stage of hypothermia – organ failure, metabolic shutdown, coma and death – can occur if the core body temperature drops from its optimum temperature of 37°C (98.6°F) to below 32.2°C (90°F). Ultra swims are rare in truly freezing waters, as over many hours hypothermia would claim even the fittest individuals. Yet temperate water temperatures of 13–18°C (55–64.5°F) can have a severe effect on physical performance, numbing muscles and reducing energy levels if the swimmer isn't familiar with the sensations.

The key is acclimatization. The Channel Swimming Association (CSA) recommends that anyone intending to do a Channel swim regularly takes cold baths and showers, and swims in the sea frequently, even during the winter months (although only for a few minutes at a time during these periods). Other cold-resistance training includes sleeping with little bed clothing and windows open during the chilly months.

Many ultra-swimmers, at least those not wearing wet suits, apply grease to their bodies. This acts as an insulator against the cold, provides limited protection against jellyfish stings and also guards against chafing at various points around the body. (Chafing is a common problem when distance swimming, given that during an ultra-marathon such as the Channel crossing a swimmer will make in the region of 45,000 strokes.) The concoctions applied to the body vary according to local recipes, but a typical mix is 50/50 Lanoline/Vaseline. The grease is obdurate stuff when applied, and the swimmer needs to ensure that although his body is coated, he does not leave any on his hands as greasy hands are less efficient at scooping through the water, and they can also deposit grease onto facemasks or goggles.

Preparation for an ultra swim, like any extreme fitness event, should begin many months prior to the actual challenge. If the water is cold, the swimmer can start small, beginning with 10–15 minute swims but adding 15 minutes to every subsequent swim. Gradually the times should build to several hours, and by three months before the event the swimmer should be able to swim solidly for seven–eight hours in the race-day sea conditions, and repeat these swims

Backstroke Crawl

During this backstroke crawl, note the wide arc taken by the arms on the upstroke and the straight alignment of next and back, both ingredients of an efficient stroke.

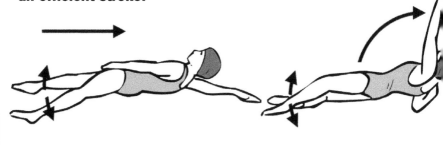

over several days. The immediate days before the race, however, should be spent in complete rest.

Swimming the Distance

Swimming marathons in open seas are gruelling in the extreme. Ingestion of salt water often makes swimmers bitterly ill, forcing them to swim through unwholesome complaints such as nausea and vomiting. The salt water can rub skin raw and cause swelling (the faces of extreme swimmers are often virtually unrecognizable at the end of their events). Debris, including oil from boat engines, can also be swallowed

if care isn't taken. Jellyfish stings are common, and sometimes support teams will have to scare off inquisitive or aggressive sharks that suddenly hone in on the limb movements of the swimmer.

Apart from all these very practical concerns, the swimmer must keep his focus on the sheer slog of repeated arm and leg movements over many hours. The technical details of specific swimming strokes will not be covered in detail here, as anyone considering an ultra swim should have already mastered the techniques. (If not, he or she should not be considering marathon swims.)

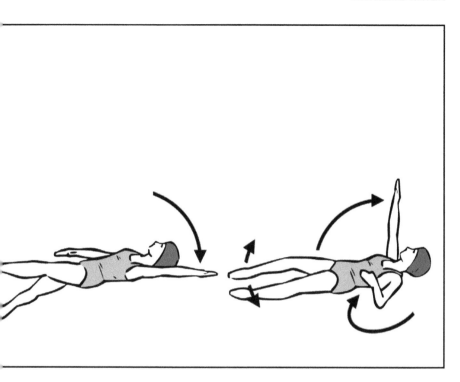

However, the essential points with any long-distance swimming stroke are that it should be both energy efficient and deliver maximum distance for every cycle of the technique. Typically, the three strokes you will use for an ultra swim are breaststroke, the crawl and sidestroke, with various types of backstroke usually reserved for either a rest or other practical purpose.

Have all your swimming techniques professionally assessed at the beginning of your training so you can iron out any bad habits early on. A critical objective is to make yourself as streamlined as possible in the water, which usually has the ancillary benefit

of reducing tension around key areas of the body – particularly the neck, back and shoulders. A slight tension can be endured for the duration of an hour in the swimming pool, but over many hours the pain can intensity until it stops the swim, or at least has a detrimental effect on your time.

Strokes

Breaststroke is the classic distance-swimming stroke, for reasons that become apparent in the U.S. Navy's swimming manual: 'breaststroke is generally considered the best survival stroke when one must swim in open water. The advantages of this

Breaststroke

**A smooth and coordinated
stroke makes the
breaststroke streamlined
and energy efficient. The
arm stroke and the leg kick
should be simultaneous.**

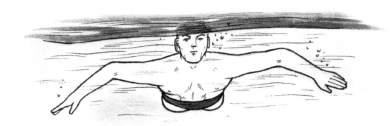

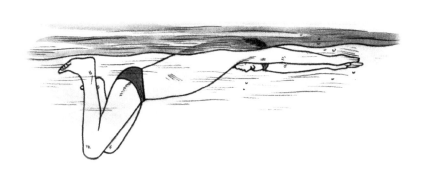

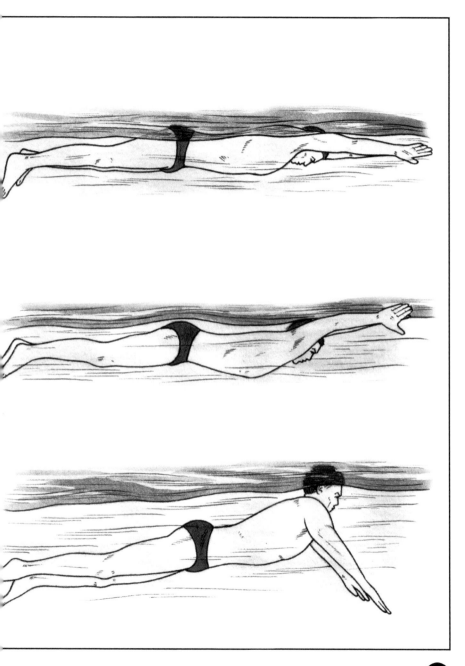

U.S. Army Tips – Surviving Shark Attacks

Stay with other swimmers. A group can maintain a 360-degree watch. A group can either frighten or fight off sharks better than one man.

Avoid urinating. If you must, only do so in small amounts. Let it dissipate between discharges. If you must defecate, do so in small amounts and throw it as far away from you as possible. Do the same if you must vomit.

If a shark attack is imminent while you are in the water, splash and yell just enough to keep the shark at bay. Sometimes yelling underwater or slapping the water repeatedly will scare the shark away. Conserve your strength for fighting in case the shark attacks.

If attacked, kick and strike the shark. Hit the shark on the gills or eyes if possible. If you hit the shark on the nose, you may injure your hand if it glances off and hits its teeth.

– FM 3-05-70, *Survival*, 16-78–16-80

stroke include good forward visibility, controlled breathing (the ability to take a breath during the trough of a wave and to return the head into the water during the crest) when swimming in choppy seas, a powerful kick while wearing boots or shoes and an efficient energy-conserving glide' (U.S. Navy, *Naval Swimmer and Instructor's Manual*, 8.3). Breaststroke's excellent seagoing characteristics means that it is worth mastering. The thrust of the legs and kick of the arms should be perfectly coordinated and powerful, and followed by a very smooth glide position, with the head down in the water and the back of the neck properly aligned with the spine. A streamlined glide position means that each power phase delivers maximum travel in the water; your breathing should also be synchronized with the beginning of the power phase, the head just lifting out of the water as the arms and legs are 'cocked' ready for the stroke.

Free-diving

Free-diving is a mental discipline that also requires formidable cardio-respiratory stamina. Incredibly, the current record for holding the breath under water exceeds 10 minutes.

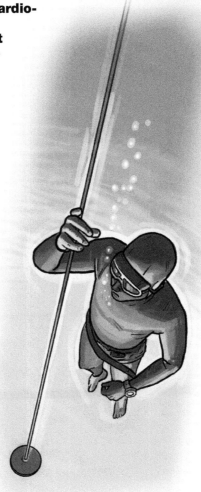

Maintaining the correct bearing is the difficult thing when swimming breaststroke in the sea. Staying close to the support boat is the most reliable mode of navigation; you can also switch to swimming on the leeward side of the boat, to provide protection against wind and spray. If any landmarks are available, however, snatched glances at them will give you some reference for maintaining the correct course.

The U.S. Navy also teaches its personnel a distinctive swimming stroke called the 'combat sidestroke'. It is situated somewhat between a crawl and a sidestroke, and has several key advantages:

The combat sidestroke is a variation of the sidestroke commonly seen with Special Warfare swimming programs. It is faster than the normal

Kayak

A kayak differs from a canoe in the position of the seat (with the rower's legs stretched out in front) and the use of a two-paddled blade.

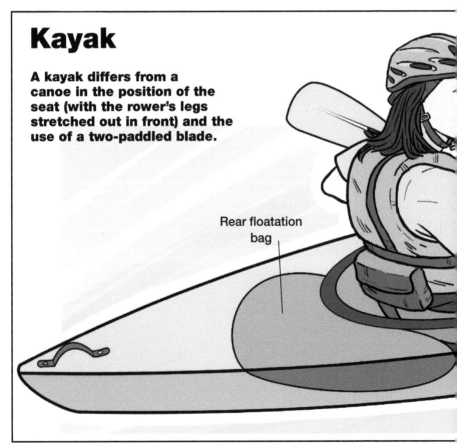

Rear floatation bag

sidestroke, offers good forward and sideward visibility, and has excellent controlled breathing when swimming in rough seas. It is identical to the normal sidestroke with exceptions being head position and breathing. During this stroke the swimmer rotates his/her head to the side and inhales during the recovery of the top arm, and then places the face into the water during the propulsion of the top arm and the propulsive phase of the kick. This breathing and head action is repeated with each stroke. The head rotation and breathing of this stroke is similar to the crawl stroke.

– U.S. Navy, *Naval Swimmer and Instructor's Manual*, 8.5

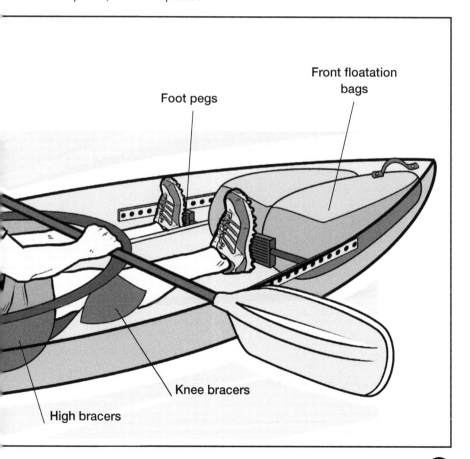

Foot pegs

Front floatation bags

Knee bracers

High bracers

Rolling a Canoe

Knowing how to right a canoe might save your life. Break the roll into stages: preparation by bracing your knees; rolling the canoe through the water by flicking your hips; and resurfacing by using your paddle to propel yourself upwards.

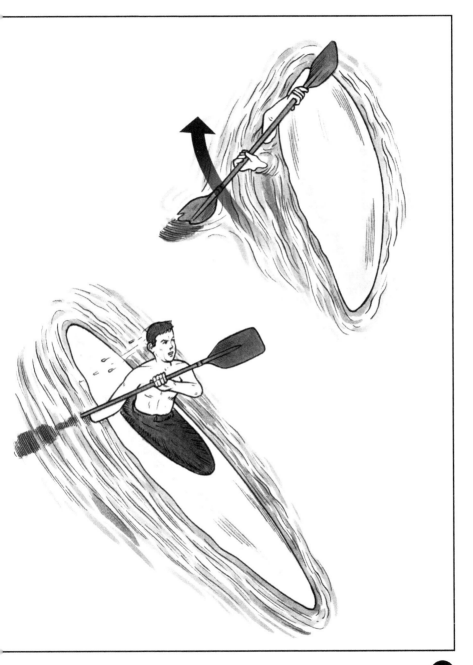

Learning the combat sidestroke is a useful addition to the endurance swimmer's box of tricks. It can give you an optional stroke to maintain progress even when the seas get rough around you. Its speed advantages over common sidestroke also mean that you can keep a strong pace. As with any new technique, you will need to become completely conversant with combat sidestroke before you can consider it part of your endurance swimming technique.

Other Aquatic Challenges

Swimming is by far the most popular aquatic endurance sport, but it is not the only one. The list of sports, if we include sailing disciplines, is too broad to cover in depth here. We can nevertheless briefly assess some of the other options for extreme fitness in water.

Free-diving

Free-diving is a blanket term for sports involving diving underwater and staying under for as long as the swimmer can hold his or her breath – no artificial breathing equipment is permitted. There are various forms of free-diving, with their own governing bodies. Some are as simple as going just beneath the water and seeing how long you can hold your breath, while more involved apnoea activities require the swimming to use a guide rope to descend to great depths (for

a human being). The five main forms of depth free-diving are free immersion, constant weight, constant weight without fins, variable weight and no limits.

The physiological data produced by free-diving is alarming and inspiring. Professional free-divers are capable of descending to depths of more than 100m (328ft), their heart rates dropping precariously low, their limbs deprived of blood by vasoconstriction, the lungs compressed dramatically (ironically, the compressed lungs can give the free-diver the sensation that they have plenty of oxygen). Strange, hypnotic mental states and blackouts can result from the oxygen deprivation – an altogether dangerous cocktail that has resulted in the deaths of several world-class free-divers.

Given the dangers of free-diving, the sport needs to be approached with caution. If you are intent on practising it, join an accredited free-diving organization and follow proven training regimes as recommended by experienced free-divers. Training has two main components: 1. Breath control; 2. Muscle control while under the effects of oxygen deprivation. The former is achieved by complex training techniques involving hyperventilation (to achieve maximum oxygenation of the blood), special breathing techniques and, of course, breath-holding for ever longer periods of time. It also requires meditative

Workout	Description
Steady state	20 to 40 minutes at a pace that barely allows you to chat with a partner
Intervals	Three to five sets of 300 to 500m [984–1640ft] at a fast pace with two minutes of rest between each set
Fartleks	Alternate one minute hard and one minute easy for 20 minutes
Long and slow	6000m [19,685ft] at an easy pace
Time trial	2000 meters [6561ft] at a record pace

– Patrick Deuster (ed.), *U.S. Navy SEAL Physical Fitness Guide*, p.44

training, teaching the mind to fight panic and overcoming the core biological urge to gulp in the air. The second component is developed through combining breath-holding with physical tasks. For example, on land the free-diver might hold his breath for one minute then walk or run as far as possible until he needs to take in air. Some people can cover distances of several hundred metres this way, with the athlete training his body to work efficiently in anaerobic conditions.

Free-diving is a growing sport, and those who master it develop extraordinary levels of physical fitness, an unequalled comfort in the water and a strangely powerful control over their mental functions. The attractions are there, but train with caution and get a full health check prior to putting your heart and lungs under such heavy strain.

Rowing
Rowing is hugely popular worldwide, partly owing to the diverse range of techniques, vessels and team configurations under the term. To be accurate, we must distinguish between rowing and paddling. Rowing involves boats in which the oars are held in place by a pivot fixed to the boat itself; in paddling sports (such as white-water rafting) the oar (singular) is not attached to the boat. Hence in rowing much of the force of propulsion comes from the legs, pushing against the oars in a sliding seat, while in paddling the force is applied primarily through the arms and shoulders.

SEAL Team Dinghy

Team rowing requires a team mindset, as you will expend valuable energy not getting anywhere if you do not work together. SEAL dinghy teams often use a leader to direct the rowing effort.

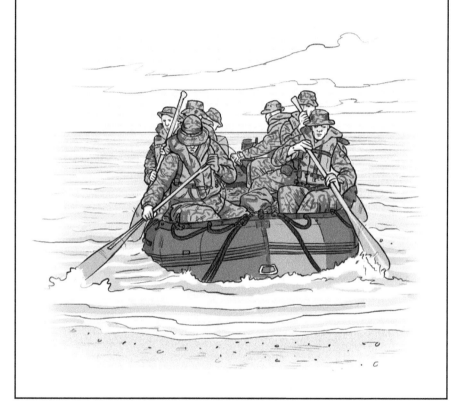

Rowing is supremely good for your physical development. Like swimming it provides a full-body workout, crafting most of the body's major muscle groups, plus it builds up cardiovascular endurance. It is also good for developing flexibility, as it puts the limbs through the full range of movement. Rowing has many endurance events to offer, both on inland waters and out at sea. In Britain, for example, there are events such as the Boston Rowing Marathon, a 50km (31 mile) race held on the third Sunday of September each year, and open to all types of rower, from crews to individuals. For those who want something altogether more challenging, there is the biannual Atlantic Rowing Race, a distance of 4700km (2930 miles) from the Canary Islands to the West Indies, a pairs race that requires superb boat technology, a lean attitude to packing supplies and round-the-clock endurance.

Special Forces Rowing

Special forces units such as the U.S. Navy SEALs also train their candidates in rowing and paddling techniques, particularly the latter in the context of amphibious deployments in inflatable boats or kayaks. The *U.S. Navy SEAL Physical Fitness Guide* also recommends static rowing machines for building up strength and endurance. (Many gyms actually hold a variety of team and individual marathon events just for rowing machines, so you don't have to get yourself wet to enjoy the full physical benefits of the sport.) The manual makes four recommendations for how you can get the most benefit from a rowing machine workout:

- *The motion of the entire stroke should be fluid*
- *A stroke rate between 24 and 30 per minute should be the goal*
- *Your grip should be loose and comfortable with wrists level*
- *The rule of thumb should be a longer not a harder workout*

– Patrick Deuster (ed.), *U.S. Navy SEAL Physical Fitness Guide*, p.43

The problem with the rowing machine, as the manual goes on to point out, is that of boredom – there is no change of view within the confines of a gym. The issue of boredom is compounded by an unvarying routine, so the manual suggests some alternative rowing workouts that provide added motivation as well enhancing your general rowing technique:

Mixed rowing training such as these workouts will provide excellent endurance building for all manner of sports, not just rowing, so is encouraged as a general training routine.

In on-water rowing, there is plenty more to think about than when seated on a rowing machine. Not only is there coordination to consider – when part of the rowing pair or team – but the rower must also navigate, cope with sea conditions and deal with the physical pressures of being exposed to the elements. You also have to keep the rhythm of the rows, no matter what the external world is throwing at you.

Rowing Technique

When performing the power stroke in rowing, thrust out with your legs before your draw the oars back with your arms.

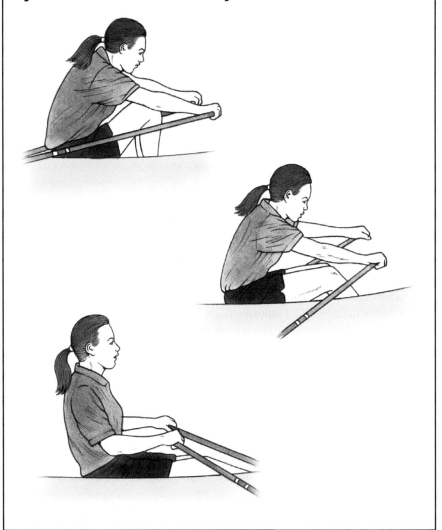

Analyzing Technique

The rule holds that if you going to take part in any sport at an extreme level, have a professional analyze your technique early on in your training to iron out any bad habits you may have picked up. There are four fundamental elements you need to focus on in any rowing sport: the catch, the drive, the finish and the recovery. The catch refers to the moment at which the blades of the oars enter the water. At this point the legs are fully bent, but to apply the drive – the power stroke – the legs are locked out straight, with the back kept in the same forward-leaning angle. The arms are also kept straight during this phase; never forget it is the legs, hips and back muscles that provide most of the power in rowing, not the arms. The finish comes at the end of the leg extension, when the rower leans back and pulls the arms into the chest (the handles should terminate at the bottom of the rib cage). The recovery phase occurs when the rower lifts the oars from the water and goes back into the catch position.

All four stages of this movement should be performed cleanly and powerfully by an endurance rower. Rowing speed can be anywhere from 20 to 50 strokes a minute, so any awkwardness in the technique will quickly be felt in muscular aches and pains. Keep the head upright and looking forward, don't shrug your shoulders during the drive and ensure that you breathe properly – exhale as you drive, inhale as you recover.

For endurance rowing, the key is to focus on maintaining the good form and a regular stroke rhythm. Erratic changes of pace are likely to tire you more, and will probably have a negative impact on your rowing times. In your training, however, you can build in pace variations to improve your fitness and muscular stamina. For example, you can separate your row into 15-minute blocks, starting the block at around 20 strokes per minute, but building up to 30 per minute for the 15th minute. Then you drop back down again and repeat the pattern. This routine trains you to apply more pressure when required. In balance, some of your training sessions should focus on long rows at 50–75 per cent of your race speed, working more on meticulous technique rather than speed.

Practice Conditions

Of course, you should make sure that you do practice sessions in the water conditions you ultimately intend to face. Get used to the rhythms of rowing through waves and against currents, and, as with open-water endurance swimming, ensure that you are not interfering with any shipping lanes or traffic. Whether you row on still waters or rough seas, the sport is virtually guaranteed to build you into a superb athlete.

Rowing Technique

This diagram shows the full sequence of rowing technique. Note how the rower compresses his legs fully prior to the power stroke, then extends them before drawing on the cable with the arms.

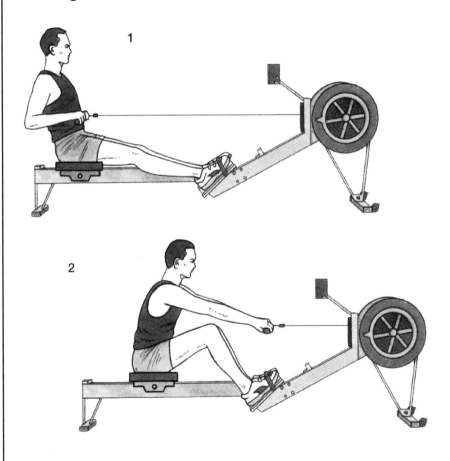

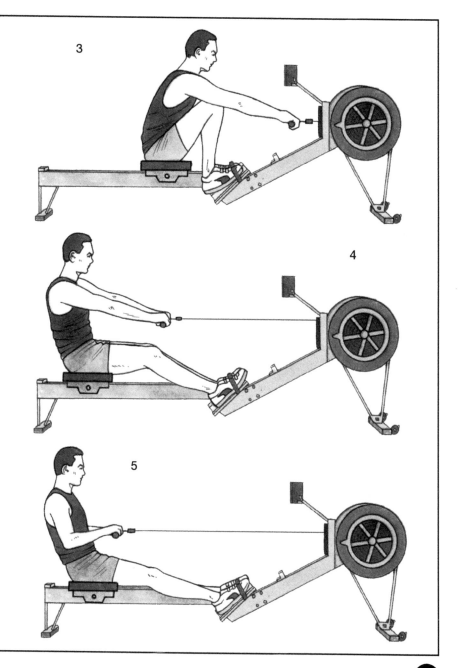

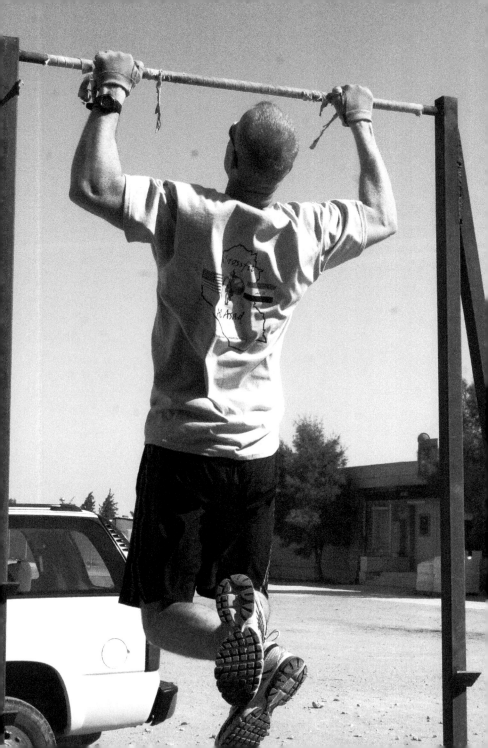

5

Strength training can be an end in itself, as demonstrated by sports such a bodybuilding and powerlifting. Yet doing weights and resistance exercises can also help improve performance in a range of other sports by developing a strong and supportive musculature.

Extreme Resistance

Strength training has long been encouraged by Special Forces units, both within its official training programmes and as an extra-curricular activity to encourage the development of physically strong warriors. It should be noted, however, that military units rarely encourage their soldiers to develop a professional bodybuilder's physique. People who sculpt their bodies into muscular works of art are undoubtedly athletes in their chosen sphere, but the bodies they create are not necessarily ideally suited to the demands of military life. For a start, although the muscle profiles are huge, large muscles doesn't equate to stamina, speed and endurance – in fact, many very large bodybuilders can quickly tire under endurance exercises, as they are attempting to transport a lot of extra weight. Furthermore, the joints of very large people – whether obese or bodybuilders – can often be weaker than those of lighter individuals.

A key distinction to be made in strength training is that between those who train for performance and those who train for shape alone. The latter will not be a focus of this chapter, as presentation bodybuilding is a distinctive area of physical development not necessarily tied to

Opposite: Building up your physical strength is as important as developing speed and stamina.

Multi-gym

A good
multi-gym
is designed
to provide
exercises
for every
key muscle
group. Plan
each session
around a
specific set of
muscles, such
as arms and
upper body,
or legs and
abdominals.

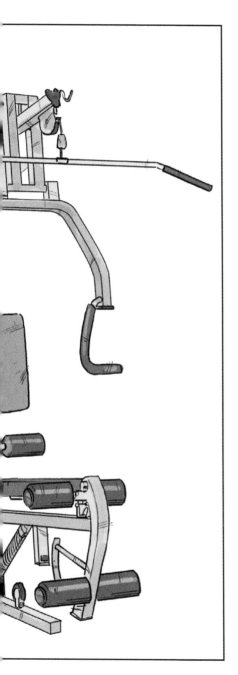

extreme fitness. Strength training for performance, however, is very much our consideration. The *Navy SEAL Fitness Guide* usefully sums up the purpose of strength training, in a military context, as the development of a musculature that supports mission objectives:

> *The focus of strength training should be its functional use for specific missions. Pure strength alone will not improve mission performance, but conversion of strength to muscle endurance should. The main objective of your strength-training program should be to increase your applied strength – an increase in applied strength will enhance your performance on physical tasks required during missions. As such, this chapter introduces concepts and practical information for achieving optimal muscle strength and endurance for job performance and prevention of injuries.*
>
> – Patrick Deuster (ed.), *Navy SEAL Fitness Guide*, p.98

The objective here of 'conversion of strength to muscle endurance' is particularly relevant to our study. Strength training, tailored to your specific requirements, will help you find new levels of applied stamina, whether your principal sport is

Bicep Curls

With the elbow on the knee, lift the weight in towards your body and back. Don't use body rocking to achieve the lift, just arm power.

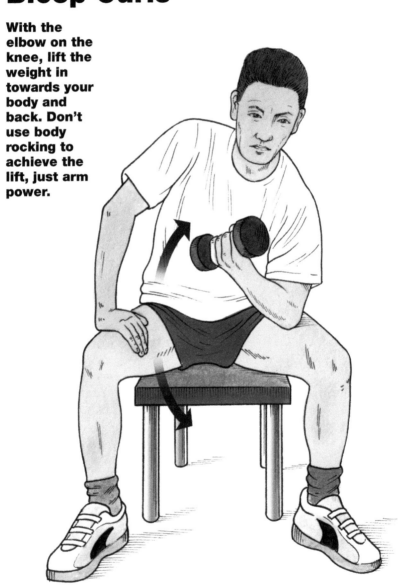

running, cycling, swimming or football. Strength training has reached the levels of such a precise art that exercises can be tailored to very specific muscle groups. Furthermore, overall muscle development usually has benefits for performance in general. If you are a runner, for example, weight training focused on the lower limbs has obvious practical applications, but building up core muscles will also provide more stability and power during a run.

Weight and resistance training is a very large subject, with a huge body of exercises. It is recommended that you join a suitable gym, with expert staff on hand, to acquire the full range of techniques available. Here we will focus on understanding the core principles of strength training and what it can contribute to your profile as an endurance athlete.

Strength without Weights

Any recruit into the armed forces will find himself, virtually from day one, regularly performing resistance exercises. Essentially, a resistance exercise is any exercise in which the muscles are put under strain against a weight or force.

A prime example would be the humble push-up. The person performing the push-up is forcing his arm, chest and back muscles to make repeated lowerings and elevations of the upper-body weight,

the number of repetitions depending on muscular strength and the type of training programme. Resistance exercises also include the activities typically performed at a weights gym, such as the bench press and dumbbell row.

Although a properly equipped gym offers excellent facilities for targeted resistance training, military training alone proves that you do not need weights to accomplish effective body strengthening and muscle development. Calisthenics – strengthening exercises using only the body weight as the source of resistance – have a long tradition of bringing soldiers to the peak of physical fitness, imbuing both stamina and strength.

Before we look at some practical calisthenics routines, a few basic concepts in resistance training need to be clarified:

Exercise – this is the specific activity being performed, such as a push-up, sit-up or squat thrust.
Repetition – refers to the individual sequence of the exercise; in a push-up, for example, a single up-and-down motion constitutes one repetition.
Set – a specified number of repetitions performed without a break is a set, e.g. 15 sit-ups
Volume – a rather less common term, 'volume' refers to the number of sets you do of an exercise, e.g. three sets of 10 push-ups.

Pull-ups

Pull-ups work the arm muscles as well as the dorsal muscles on each side of the centre of the back.

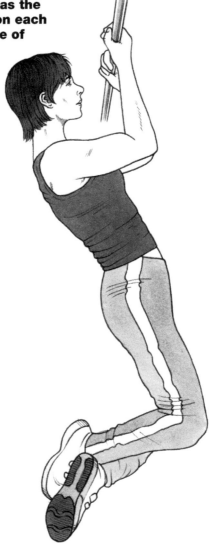

The Bent-leg Raise

Lying in the Starting Position for the sit-up, place the fingers of both hands underneath the small of the back. Raise the feet off of the ground until both the hips and knees are flexed to 90 degrees. Next, contract the abdominals as if you are preparing for a blow to the stomach. Another way to perform this drawing-in manoeuvre is to imagine pulling the navel toward the spine. Think about the amount of pressure on your fingers created by the contraction of your abdominals. Maintain the same degree of pressure as you slowly straighten the legs. As soon as you can no longer maintain the same degree of pressure on your fingers, bring the legs back to the Starting Position and repeat until one minute has elapsed.

– U.S. Army, *Army Pocket Physical Training Guide*, p.30

Rest – a period of time left for recovery between each set.

Effective calisthenics, indeed weight training in general, relies on a disciplined training programme involving deliberate and controlled progression in the repetitions and sets of a variety of exercises. You have several options for the way you control this progression. First, you can define your set by a specific time limit; for example, you might define a set as the amount of push-ups you can do in 15 seconds. To increase the level of training you can then either attempt to do more push-ups in the same amount of time, or simply increase the amount of time you spend doing push-ups. You could also increase the number of sets. Another option for progression is to increase, over time, the number of repetitions per set you perform. For example, in week one of your training programme you might perform three sets of 20 push-ups, increasing it to 25 reps in week two, 30 reps in week three and so on.

Progressive Development

You can obviously create a mix of strategies to add more interest and effect to your routine. In all resistance training, doing the same exercises to the same level of intensity week after week will

Bent-leg Raise

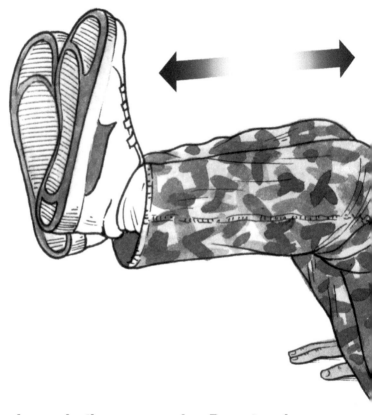

This exercise works the core muscles. Repeat each movement as slowly as possible, curling the upper back up slightly to isolate the abdominals.

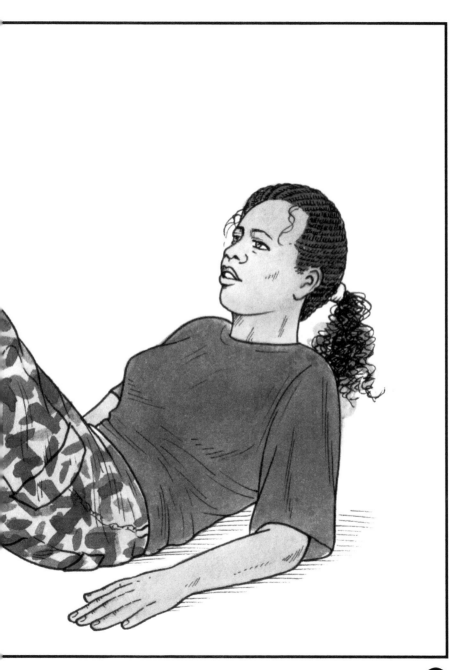

eventually result in a plateau in your improvement. Why this is so requires a basic understanding of how resistance training in general leads to increased strength and muscle mass. When you overload your muscles – i.e. put them under extreme stress – micro-tears occur in the muscle tissue. It then repairs itself, but in the process of repair it strengthens to adjust to the new loads placed upon it. This continual process of breakdown and repair is the primary mechanism of strength development.

However, the body will eventually adjust to the level of strain placed upon it, hence if you keep performing the same exercise to the same volume the muscular development will plateau and not increase. This is why resistance training has to be progressive, the increasing loads 'shocking' the body into further levels of power. The same effect can be achieved by performing new types of exercise, ones to which the body is not accustomed.

Calisthenics

Thankfully, the world of calisthenics is replete with literally dozens of exercises of varying levels of difficulty and challenge. They not only include old favourites such as push-ups, pull-ups and sit-ups, but also muscle-crunching exercises with unfamiliar names such as the windmill, flutter kick, the engine and the cross-country skier. The specific techniques of these exercises are widely available online, with excellent examples being available in the *U.S. Army's Field Manual* FM 21-20 (see www.apft-standards.com/files/fm21_20.pdf). When learning these techniques – and any weight training exercise – it is vital that you learn proper form. Perform any rep completely, going through the full range of movement and keeping the body in correct posture throughout, particularly the spine and neck. If you find that failing strength is causing collapsing form, stop the exercise, recover, then attempt to perform it again, possibly with fewer reps to enable you to keep good form.

Calisthenics routines are best performed when arranged into a circuit, a sequence of exercises performed at various 'stations'. (Note that the stations don't actually need to be in different parts of a room or field – they can actually be performed in the same place.) The type of circuit you can devise is virtually limitless, but for best results you should give each circuit a certain 'theme', and change these themes during the week's training. The themes can be designed to enhance muscle groups used in a particular sport, but to get the best out of your circuit make sure that the exercises aren't all focused on one part of the body. For example, if you want to improve your upper-body fitness for rowing, concentrating on

Tricep Lifts

Tricep lifts develop power in the shoulders, biceps and triceps. Keep the movements smooth, and lower your body until the arms are bent at 90 degrees.

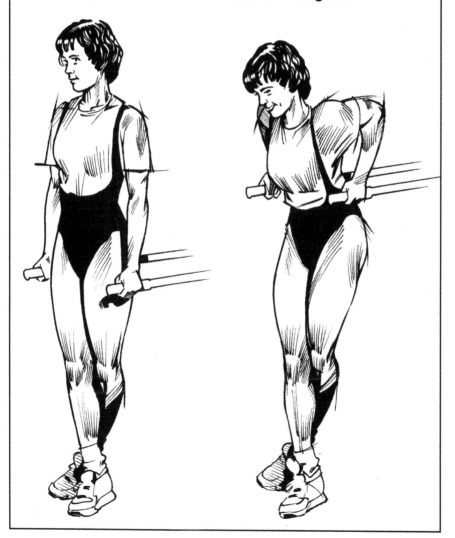

Sit-ups

From your start position of lying on the floor, bring your head and knees together so they almost touch. Alternate this technique with meeting opposite elbows to opposite knees. Keeping your hands placed softly on your head will prevent you pulling the neck.

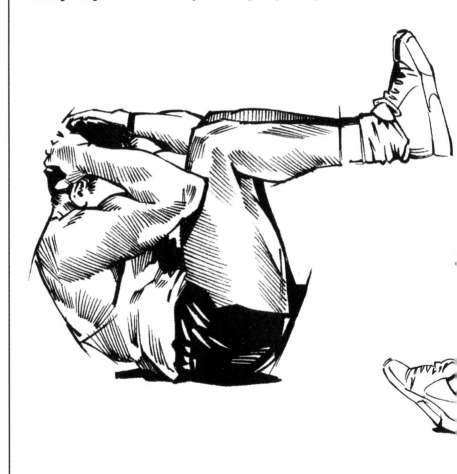

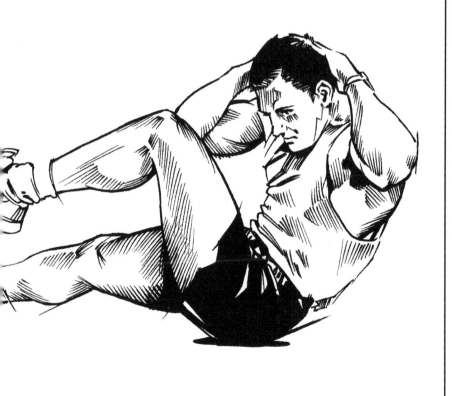

Circuit Training

A classic eight-step circuit training routine.

the arms, shoulders, back and core, a good circuit might look like this:

Station 1   – push-ups (60 secs)
              – Rest 30 secs
Station 2   – crunches (60 secs)
              – Rest 30 secs

Station 3   – burgees (60 secs)
              – Rest 30 secs
Station 4   – star jumps (60 secs)
              – Rest 30 secs
Station 5   – sprints (60 secs)
              – Rest 30 secs

Station 6 – Tricep dips (60 secs)
– Rest 30 secs
Station 7 – pull-ups (60 secs)
– Rest 30 secs
Station 8 – lunges (60 secs)
– Rest 30 secs
Station 9 – level 1 drills (one
set: 8 push-ups;
8 alternate leg squat
thrusts) (60 secs)

– Rest 30 secs
Station 10 – swimmer (60 secs)
– Rest 30 secs
Station 11 – wide-arm push-ups
(60 secs)
– Rest 30 secs
Station 12 – parallel bar dip
– Rest 60 secs
(Repeat three times)
The weighting of this circuit is towards

U.S. Army Tip – the High Jumper

Purpose: This exercise reinforces correct jumping and landing, stimulates balance and coordination, and develops explosive strength.
Starting Position: forward-leaning stance.
Cadence: MODERATE.

Count: 1. Swing arms forward and jump a few inches.
2. Swing arms backward and jump a few inches.
3. Swing arms forward and vigorously overhead while jumping.
4. Repeat Count 2. On the last repetition, return to the
Starting Position.

Check Points:
At the Starting Position, the shoulders, the knees and the balls of the feet should form a straight vertical line.
On Count 1, the arms are parallel to the ground.
On Count 3, the arms should be extended fully overhead. The trunk and legs should also be in line. On each landing, the feet should be directed forward and maintained at shoulder distance apart. The landing should be 'soft' and proceed from balls of the feet to the heels. The vertical line from the shoulders through the knees to the balls of the feet should be demonstrated on each landing.

– U.S. Army, *Army Pocket Physical Training Guide*, pp.49–50

Pull-ups with Extra Weight

When you can successfully do several sets of pull-up reps, you increase the resistance by adding weights to increase muscle development.

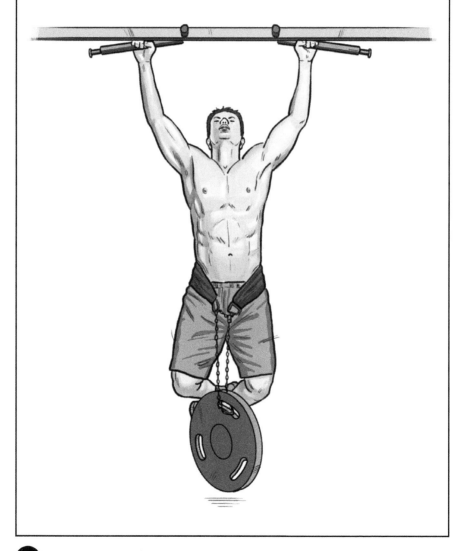

upper-body and core exercises. Doing these alone, however, would result in near-certain muscle failure for all but the super-fit, so exercises like the star jumps, shuttle sprints and lunges provide a form of physical break for the upper body, while adding their own contribution to overall fitness.

More about creating effective circuits is discussed in the next chapter. Suffice to say here that calisthenics are an ideal route to developing your body without the need for advanced gym equipment. Yet there is no denying that a well-equipped gym can deliver powerful results when approached with discipline and commitment.

Weight Training

One of the key debates in the world of weight training is the relative benefit of weights machines versus free weights. A shortcut through this debate is to

Powerlifting

Safe powerlifting requires a direct vertical alignment between the grip hands and the shoulders. Keep the neck in a natural, forward-looking position.

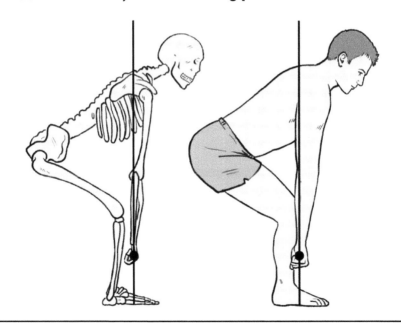

say that both have pros and cons, and therefore both can be used profitably. Some more detailed explanation is nevertheless required if you are going to get the most out of a modern gym.

Free Weights

Among many professional bodybuilders and athletes, free weights are undeniably king. One immediate advantage is that while good-quality weights machines are expensive and take up lots of space, a set of dumbbells, a bar bell and a foldaway weights bench can be picked up relatively cheaply, enabling you to create your own basic gym in most rooms. In a professional gym, you will have racks of free weights to choose from, plus other types of free-weight devices such as medicine balls and kettlebells, enabling you to get creative with a range of exercises.

The central benefit of free weights is that they work more of the intended muscle groups because you not only can go through a fuller range of motion (many weights machines have range-of-motion limitations), but you also have to work harder to stabilize

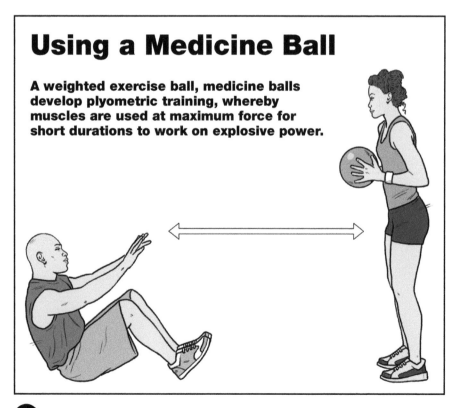

Using a Medicine Ball

A weighted exercise ball, medicine balls develop plyometric training, whereby muscles are used at maximum force for short durations to work on explosive power.

Bar Bell Lifts

Holding the bar bell at
shoulder height with your
palms facing forwards,
extend the arms upwards
until at full stretch. Hold
this position for a few
seconds before returning
to the start position and
repeating. Do not lock
your elbows.

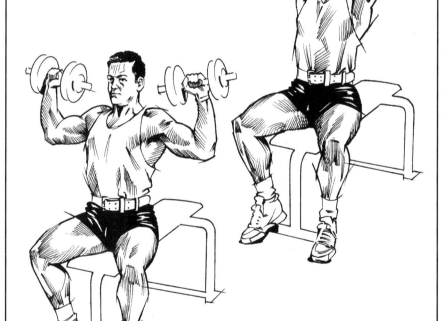

Kettle Bell Exercises

Developed in Russia, kettle bell training is good for strength and flexibility, as well as giving you a cardio workout.

Dead lift

Figure
of eight

Half get-up

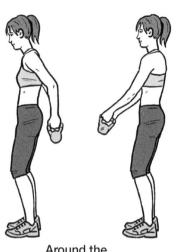

Around the
body pass

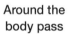

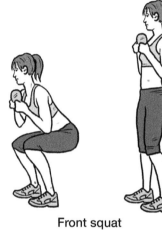

Front squat

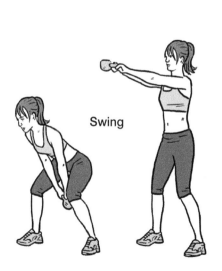

Swing

Concentrated Bicep Curl

Starting with the bar bell held low in front of you, position your arm against the curl bench for support. Perform the curl very slowly, focusing on keeping everything motionless but the arm action.

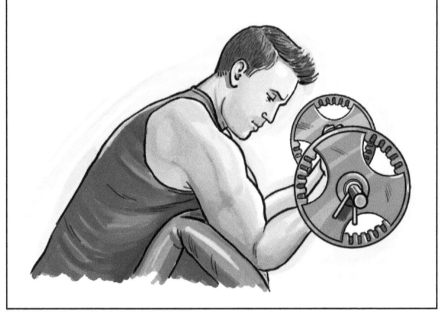

yourself through the technique. By activating your 'stabilizing' muscles, your body develops more roundly, with greater strength in the core. For those training to enhance their physique for other sports, free weights enable you to create bespoke exercises that work your muscles through functional movements. The variations are almost limitless, especially if you add kettlebells into the mix. For example, a regular forward lunge is transformed into a thigh-enhancing and core-building routine by holding a 12 or 16kg (26 or 35lb) kettlebell above your head.

Near-endless variation, a more rounded muscular development and their relative cheapness make free weights a natural choice for many. On the debit side, free weights

Dead Lifts

When dead lifting, note the grip on the bar bell uses one underhand and one overhand grip. This help you maintain balance when lifting.

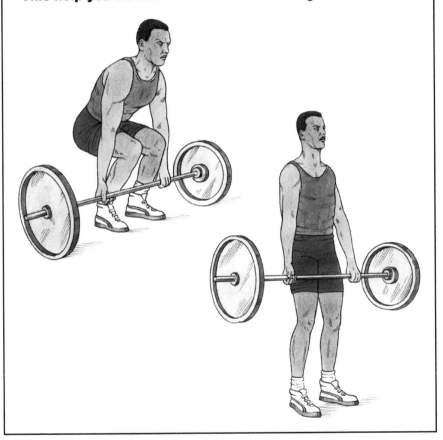

exercises are harder to perform 'cleanly' than weights machine exercises, and you will likely have to work with lower weights and progress more slowly than you would on the machines. Try to rush things and free weights are far more likely to injure you. Furthermore, many free weights exercises should only be performed safely with a spotter, who can be ready to rescue you from the weight when and if you reach the point of muscle failure. However, the need to have someone else there can be a problem for many who want to train alone.

Weights Machines

Weights are designed to work specific muscle groups with scientific precision. For example, the ever-popular lat pull-down targets the Latissimum dorsi (hence the machine's name) and a group of other muscles that surround the shoulder girdle. Weights machines tend to be extremely easy to use – the configuration of the machine in many ways dictates that you apply correct technique – but the downside of this is that you can put yourself at more risk of overloading and strain injuries. Conversely, because a weights machine doesn't require you to have the assistance of a spotter, you can perform intense resistance exercises more safely than if you were alone with some hefty free weights.

If your goal is primarily to bulk up certain aspects of your physique, weights machines can be one of the most direct routes of doing so. The muscle targeting offered by weights machines also means that you can work on muscles that you feel need specific strengthening. This advantage is also useful if you are recovering from injury and want to work vulnerable muscles in a

controlled manner, or avoid certain muscles being overworked while continuing your strength training.

Weights machines nevertheless don't strengthen the stabilizing muscles mentioned previously, so used on their own they would not produce the rounded muscular strength offered by a free weights programme.

Key Principles

As we can see, there is no knockout argument in the free weights versus weights machines debate. I would argue that the debate doesn't really need to exist in the first place, unless you are really going all out to be a professional bodybuilder, as a combination of both in your routine is both practical and useful, depending on your requirements. Just be aware of the limitations and possibilities of both forms of training.

Whatever form of exercise you do in the gym, form is everything. Occasionally you will see competitive spirits in the gym jerking huge weights into the air, their backs and shoulders flexing wildly as they run through the reps (indicating that they are using momentum as much as body strength to lift the weights). Poor technique such as this leads to injury. The U.S. Navy SEALs are very aware that its ultra-athletic personnel can spend much time in the gym. They provide some solid guidance about how to train safely:

Power Rack

The power rack is useful for practising extreme resistance training safely, as bar catchers can be fitted to prevent you being injured by falling weights.

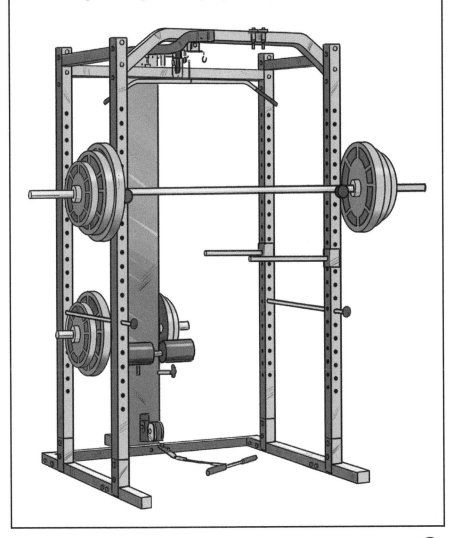

Don't concentrate all your time and energy in the weight room. It is not necessary to add mass to benefit from strength training. Proper lifting aids in injury prevention. Take care to lift properly to avoid injuries caused by lifting. You should follow a well-designed and properly supervised program for general strength.

You can occasionally perform a second set to provide additional training stimulus, but in most cases one set is sufficient to produce significant increases in strength. Perform a single set using a weight that cannot be lifted more than 8–12 times giving maximal effort and using proper technique. Generally perform 8–12 exercises per session. Move from one exercise to the next quickly, only resting the amount of time it takes to set up the proper weight at the next station. This promotes overall intensity and some cardiorespiratory adaptations. Use a split routine of upper body and lower body exercises on alternate days.

– www.sealswcc.com/navy-seals-strength-training.aspx#.UhuY-T-kbIU

The message that 'proper lifting aids in injury prevention' is the maxim of weight training. Proper technique means that you move through the full range of motion (ROM) assigned to each exercise, relying mainly on the muscles specifically targeted and avoiding any ballistic motions in an attempt to drive the weight.

Gymnastic Hoops

Excellent for weight-free resistance training, hoops also allow you to work on flexibility and range of movement.

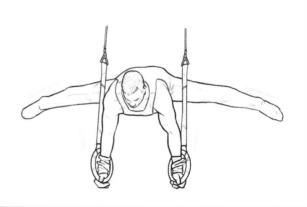

Seated Pull-downs

Working the arms, dorsal muscles and shoulders, pull-downs must be performed with a straight back and neck.

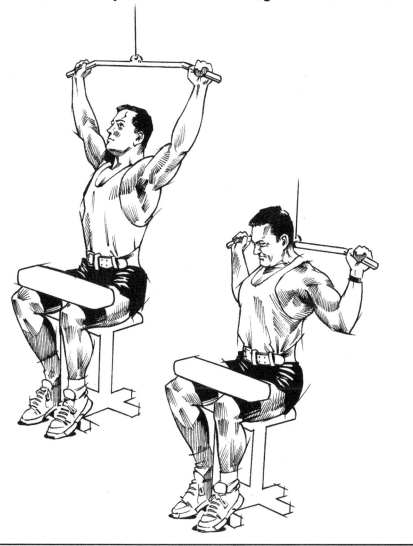

Military Weight Training

Forces personnel build regular weight training into their exercise routines, as it enhances their ability to carry weapons and packs.

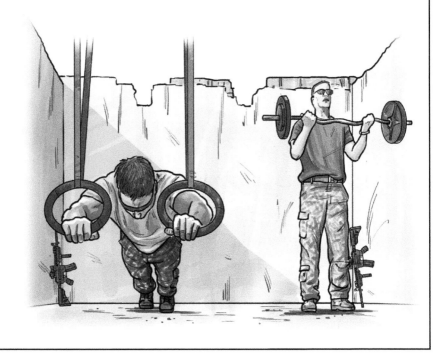

A correct number of reps is that at which you struggle to perform the last rep, but you are still able to keep good form throughout. By the last rep in the last set, you should be at the point of muscle failure. In terms of the number of reps you perform, the recommendation of 8–12 is sound. Generally, most gym experts recommend about 8–10 reps with a very heavy weight for muscle expansion, and 10–12 reps with a lighter weight (but still working to muscle failure) for more general strength and muscular endurance. This division into bulking/toning isn't quite as watertight as is often described, however. More important

Bench Presses

Note that arms should be fully extended and locked when bench pressing. Always perform bench presses with a partner to spot you.

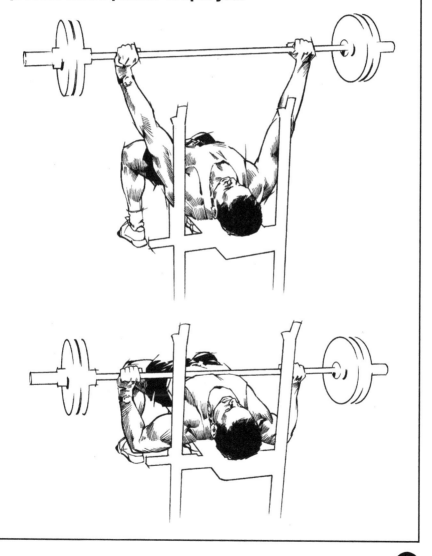

U.S. Navy Tip – Determining Repetition Maximums (RM)

The purpose of knowing your RM is to allow you to adjust the exercise intensity. As a safety measure, it is best to start out by determining your 5RM. To do this, you should not have any strenuous activity on the day of the test, and you should be properly warmed up. A spotter should always be available when conducting this test. Free weights are the recommended form of weight for this test.

Select a weight you know is light enough for 10 repetitions.
Perform 10–15 repetitions with that weight.

Rest for two minutes.
Increase weight 2–10 per cent, depending on difficulty of previous set.
Perform 6–8 repetitions.

Rest for two minutes.
Increase weight 2–10 per cent, depending on difficulty of previous set.

Rest for three minutes.
Perform 5 repetitions – this should be close to your 5RM.

– U.S. Navy, *Navy SEAL Fitness Guide*, p.98

is that you perform the reps powerfully and with control.

In terms of the routine you develop for gym weights, again the possibilities are endless. In the advice given by the SEALs above, it discusses just one set of reps per exercise, moving quickly on to the next. This creates a form of gym circuit, and can be a sharp way to achieve results, generating strength alongside cardiovascular fitness.

An example of such a circuit, one that provides an overall body workout, is as follows:
Station 1 – leg press, 8–12 reps
Station 2 – leg raise, 8–12 reps
Station 3 – leg extension, 8–12 reps
Station 4 – leg curl, 8–12 reps
Station 5 – heel raise, 8–12 reps
Station 6 – bench press, 8–12 reps
Station 7 – seated row, 8–12 reps
Station 8 – military press, 8–12 reps
Station 9 – lat pull down, 8–12 reps

Standing Bar Lift

Lifting the bar bell to just under your chin and holding it briefly gives your arms, shoulders and core muscles an effective workout.

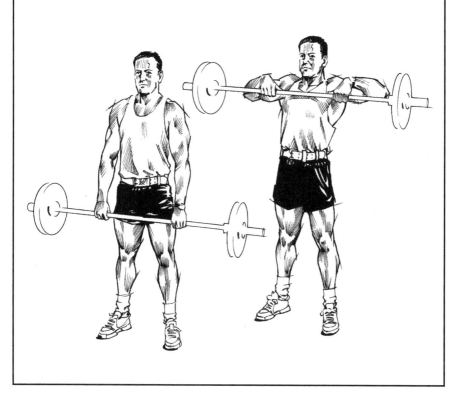

Station 10 – shrug, 8–12 reps
Station 11 – triceps extension, 8–12 reps
Station 12 – biceps curl, 8–12 reps

For many, however, the gym workout is more about strengthening than increasing stamina, and therefore follows a less frenetic path around the weights. In this case, two or three sets per exercise, with a good minute or so of rest between each set, is a sound plan. Doing this you might find that you start

Chest	Shoulders	Back	Quadri-ceps	Ham-strings	Biceps	Triceps
Flat dumbbell flys	Arnold press	Chest supported barbell or dumbell rows	Leg press	Barbell or dumbell Romanian deadlifts	Cable curls	Skull crushers
Incline barbell or dumb-bell bench press	Barbell dumb-ell or machine upright rows	Chest supported machine rows	Machine squat/ hack squat	Bar-bell or dumb-bell straight leg deadlifts	Biceps curl machine	Over-head bar-bell or dumb-bell triceps exten-sions
Decline bar-bell or dumb-bell bench press	Dumb-bell, cable or machine lateral raises	Inverted rows	Leg ex-tensions	Bar-bell or dumb-bell sumo deadlifts	Hammer curls	Flat close grip bench press
Flat chest press machine	Seated over-head bar-bell or dumb-bell press	Barbell dumb-bell or machine shrugs	Bar-bell or dumb-bell squats	Cable pull throughs	Concen-tration curls	Decline close grip bench press

The above is a list, not exhaustive, of good weights exercises for targeting major muscle groups.

Chest	Shoulders	Back	Quadri-ceps	Ham-strings	Biceps	Triceps
Incline chest press machine	Standing over-head bar-bell or dumb-bell	T-bar rows	Bar-bell or dumb-bell front squats	Good morn-ings	Standing bar-bell or dumb-bell curls	Close grip push-ups
Decline chest press machine	Over-head machine press	Seated cable rows	Bar-bell or dumb-bell squats	Leg curls	Bar-bell or dumb-bell preacher curls	Laying bar-bell or dumb-bell triceps exten-sions
Flat bar-bell or dumb-bell bench press	Dumb-bell, cable or machine front raises	Lat pull-downs	Bar-bell or dumb-bell lunges	Cable pull throughs	Seated dumb-bell curls	Cable press downs
Incline dumb-bell flys	Barbell dumb-bell or machine rear delt rows, raises or flys	Bent over bar-bell or dumb-bell rows		Good morn-ings	Incline dumb-bell curls	Bench dips
Decline dumb-bell flys						

Quad Squats

Stretching out the muscles you used during resistance training is important for avoiding pain and injury. The quad squat, or lunge, strengthens the supporting leg while stretching the hamstrings of the extended leg.

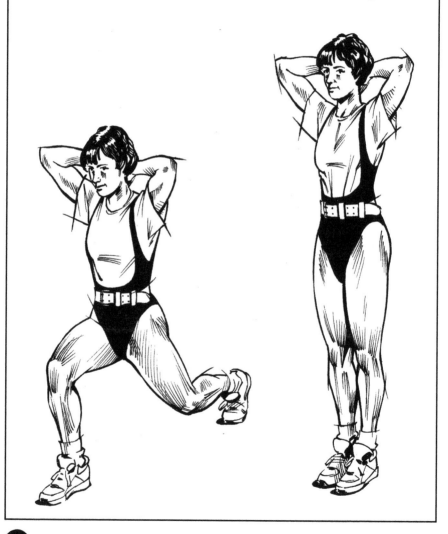

to struggle sooner into the reps as you go through the sets. So, while you might be able to do a full set of 12 reps with good form in the first set, by Set 3 you are struggling after Rep 5. In this case, reduce the weight and complete the full set, even if it means going down to what you consider embarrassingly low weights.

If you visit you gym about two or three times a week, it makes sense to configure each session to specific muscle sets, such as chest, back and arms for one session, then legs and core for the next. Mixing it up like this ensures that one group of intensively worked muscles has time to heal and strengthen before putting them under heavy loads again.

Get your gym instructor to show you these core techniques, and make them your own. Add a well-crafted weights training programme to an endurance sport and you have the perfect combination for reaching your peak levels of fitness. Weights training can lead to an impressively shaped and powerful-looking physique. It can also provide substantial long-term health benefits, such as strong joints and bones, fat-burning and more injury-resistant muscles.

British Army Tips – Core Development Exercises

Dorsal Raise
- Lie on your front with hands by temples
- Use your lower back muscles to lift your shoulders and chest off the floor
- Lift slowly; do not bounce off the floor

Assisted Sit-up
- Lie back with knees bent and ankles supported
- Hold your arms across your chest
- Keep your shoulders back and neck straight
- Brace your abdomen and sit all the way up
- Lower yourself under control
- Do not allow your shoulders to touch the floor

www.army.mod.uk/documents/general/Fitnes_LowRes.pdf

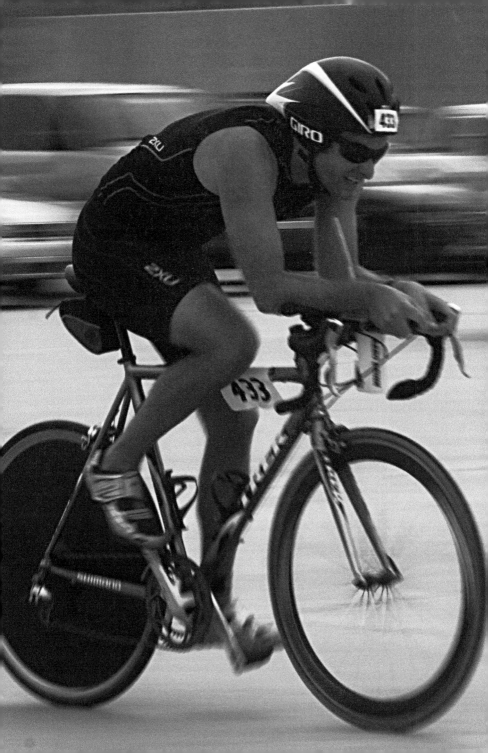

Cross-training comes naturally to Special Forces. High-level military operations require soldiers with a flexible type of fitness, one that can switch from rowing an inflatable craft into shore then switching to a long overland advance, all the while handling heavy loads of pack and weaponry. The multi-faceted fitness required to perform such feats is beyond the remit of just one sporting activity, hence the physical training instructors must apply a variety of methods to achieve the right results. This mixed training regime is known as cross-training.

All sporting activities benefit from the practice of cross-training, but some absolutely depend on it. The ultimate example is the triathlon, an almost unsurpassed test of all-round stamina and endurance. Triathlons are composed of three back-to-back stamina events – swimming, running and cycling – arranged in various distances. At the extremes of triathlon is the internationally renowned 'iron man' event, which consists of a 3.8km (2.4 miles) swim, 180.2km (112 miles) bike ride and a full marathon run of 42.2km (26.2 miles). Needless to say, only a tenacious few are capable of such a test. More about the tactics and training related to triathlons is discussed below.

• •

Opposite: Cross-training is a good method for alleviating boredom and remaining fully motivated.

6

Cross-training can be the ultimate development strategy for the serious athlete. By training in several contrasting activities, an endurance sportsman will take himself to new levels of physical achievement.

Mixing It Up

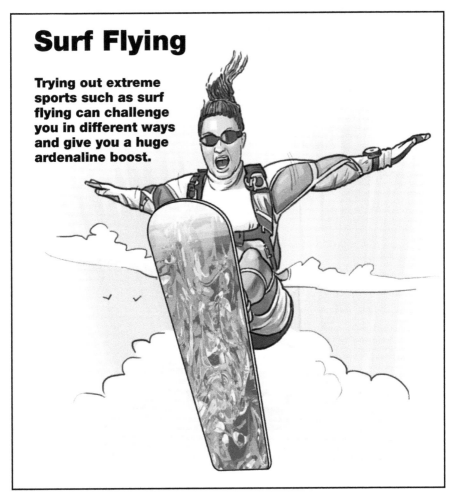

Surf Flying

Trying out extreme sports such as surf flying can challenge you in different ways and give you a huge ardenaline boost.

First, we will look at some of the fundamentals of cross-training and how they can be built into your own sporting life.

Sporting Choices

Cross-training does need a certain degree of self-control. Some people attempt to incorporate too many sports within their training programme, often resulting in over-training or a lack of focus on a core activity. Roughly speaking, two or three different activities are the maximum someone can fit into an otherwise busy life. You should attempt to seek balance in your cross-training, so that the activities

Rock Climbing

Rock climbing produces flexibility and immensely powerful limbs, as well as testing intelligence and mental control.

you choose both complement and contrast with one another. For example, a cross-training programme that consists of running, weight training and badminton sensibly incorporates aerobic, anaerobic and strength-building activities for all-round fitness. A programme of running, badminton and tennis, however, includes two similar activities. This mix might be driven by social considerations – not a bad thing, but not the best way to enhance physical performance.

There are some individual sporting activities, however, that within themselves incorporate an aspect of cross-training. In the military world, an excellent example of this is one of the central pillars of physical training – obstacle courses.

Testing Motor Skills

The obstacle course, configured in a challenging manner, is a powerful trial even to those of athletic prowess. The thinking behind this form of physical training is spelt out in the U.S. Army's *Physical Fitness Training Manual:* 'Physical performance and success in combat may depend on a soldier's ability to perform skills like those required on the obstacle course. For this reason, and because they help develop and test basic motor skills, obstacle courses are valuable for physical training' (U.S. Army, FM 21-20, 8-1). The rationale given here suggests that the obstacle course produces rounded fitness that has as much application in a physically vigorous daily life as it does for sporting activities. A properly designed obstacle course can take anything from a few minutes to more than an hour to complete, but it will test stamina, upper- and lower-body strength, flexibility, mind-body coordination, core resilience and mental commitment.

The aforementioned U.S. Army field manual roughly places obstacle courses into two categories:

There are two types of obstacle courses – conditioning and confidence. The conditioning course has low obstacles that must be negotiated quickly. Running the course can be a test of the soldier's basic motor skills and physical condition. After soldiers receive instruction and practice the skills, they run the course against time. A confidence course has higher, more difficult obstacles than a conditioning course. It gives soldiers confidence in their mental and physical abilities and cultivates their spirit of daring. Soldiers are encouraged, but not forced, to go through it. Unlike conditioning courses, confidence courses are not run against time.

– U.S. Army, FM 21-20, 8-1
Most endurance athletes will

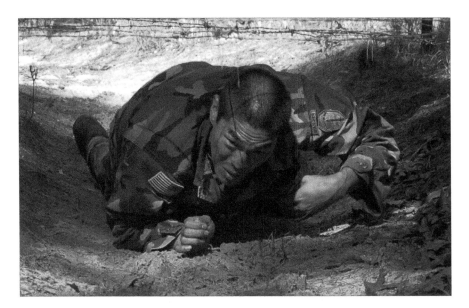

When performing crawling exercises, establish a strong rhythm with the elbows and knees and keep looking forward.

readily identify with the conditioning obstacle course. The types of obstacles within a conditioning course are highly variable. A good course will feature some 20–25 different obstacles, each separated by about 20m (64ft) of space that can be crossed at a sprint. The obstacles will test all parts of the musculature. Based on military design guidelines, typical obstacles include:

Jumping Obstacles
- Ditch/trench
- Hurdles
- Platform

Dodging/Coordination Obstacles
- Diagonal lanes
- Mazes
- Log lattices
- Tyre runs

Vertical Climbing and Surmounting Obstacles
- Climbing rope
- Cargo net
- Climbing wall
- Climbing pole

Horizontal Traversing Obstacles
- Monkey bars
- Horizontal pipe or beam
- Rope

Jumping Obstacles

When performing any
jumping obstacle,
land with 'soft' knees,
bending them prior to
impact and deepening
the bend to act like a
car's shock absorber.

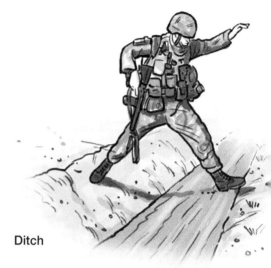

Ditch

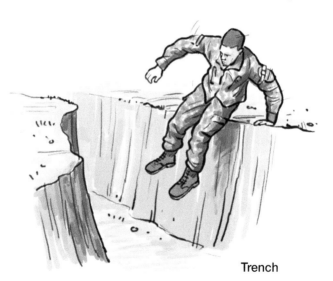

Trench

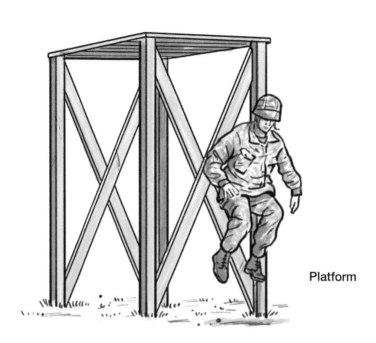

Platform

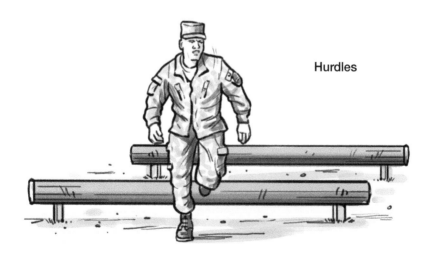

Hurdles

Log Carrying Drill

Log carrying drills build group cohesion and camaraderie. Practice switching shoulders in a coordinated fashion and at regular timed intervals.

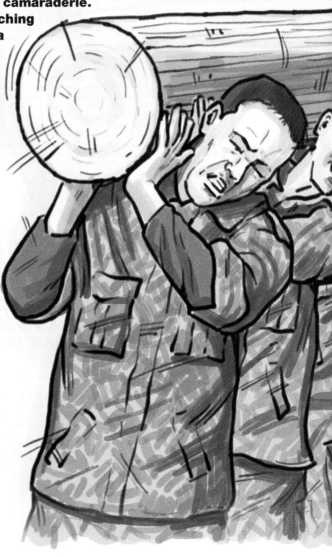

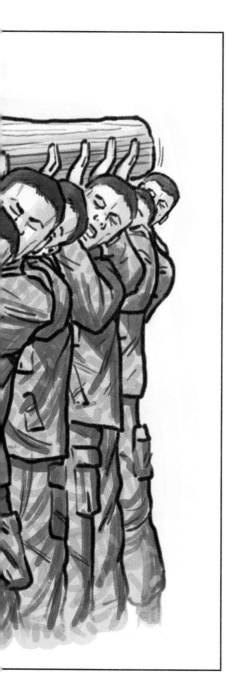

Crawling Obstacles
- Wire
- Tunnel
- Low rail

Vaulting Obstacles
- Beam
- Fence
- Low wall
- Rope swing

Balancing Obstacles
- Log
- Beam

This list is not exhaustive. Obstacle courses can include other unusual challenges such as log carries, island hoppers (jumping between isolated circular platforms) or inverted rope descents, or include calisthenic exercises between the various obstacle stations. The only limit to the nature of the course is the imagination of the designer.

Introduce yourself gently to obstacle courses. By virtue of their design they can be dangerous facilities, presenting the risk of twisting, impact and falling injuries. Get used to the nature of the obstacles before attempting to establish or smash a good time. Take special care that on any jumping obstacles you land properly, striking the ground with both your feet and bending your knees strongly to absorb the shock. If you are feeling exhausted, pause briefly before

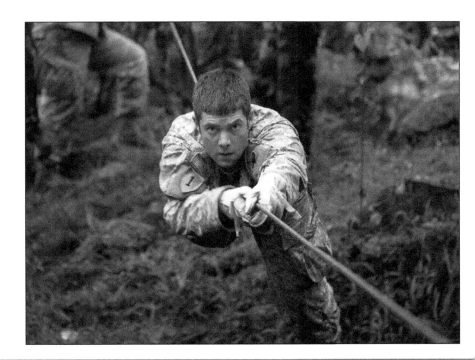

U.S. Military Obstacle – Inverted Rope Descent

Soldiers climb the tower, grasp the rope firmly and swing their legs upward. They hold the rope with their legs to distribute the weight between their legs and arms. Braking the slide with their feet and legs, they proceed down the rope. Soldiers must be warned that they may get rope burns on their hands. This obstacle can be dangerous when the rope is slippery. Soldiers leave the rope at a clearly marked point of release. Only one soldier at a time is allowed on the rope. Soldiers should not shake or bounce the ropes. This obstacle requires two instructors – one on the platform and the other at the base.

– U.S. Army, FM 21-20, 8-1

Opposite: When making a rope crossing, use the dangling lower leg as a pendulum-like aid to balance. Look ahead at all times.

stepping onto any balancing obstacle, to control your breathing and focus on the switch from fast movement to slow balance.

The U.S. military gives excellent advice for the correct attitude for preparing and tackling obstacle courses safely:

Units should prepare their soldiers to negotiate obstacle courses by doing conditioning exercises beforehand. Soldiers should attain an adequate level of conditioning before they run the confidence course. Soldiers who have not practiced the basic skills or run the conditioning course should not be allowed to use the confidence course. Instructors must explain and demonstrate

Belaying

Used for safety during rock climbing, belaying breaks the fall by securing supports to the rock and applying friction to the rope.

Abseiling

Abseiling or rappelling is the rapid descent down a rock face. This is useful practice for soldiers, as troops can be deployed by abseiling from a moving helicopter if there are no safe landing zones available.

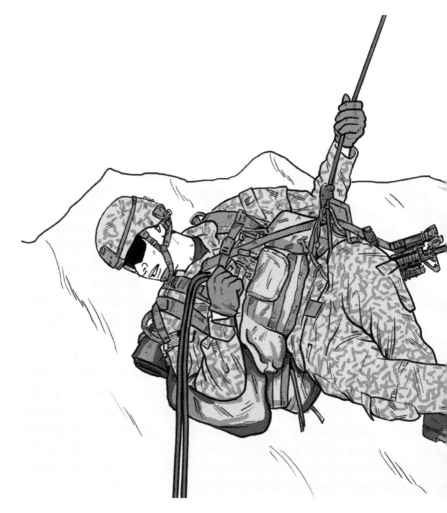

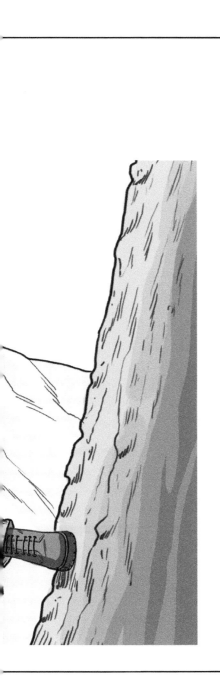

the correct ways to negotiate all obstacles before allowing soldiers to run them. Assistant instructors should supervise the negotiation of higher, more dangerous obstacles. The emphasis is on avoiding injury. Soldiers should practice each obstacle until they are able to negotiate it. Before they run the course against time, they should make several slow runs while the instructor watches and makes needed corrections. Soldiers should never be allowed to run the course against time until they have practiced on all the obstacles.
– U.S. Army, FM 21-20, 8-1

Once you become confident, however, you can obviously go for it, trying to establish self-assured, rhythmic movement through every type of obstacle and really applying the speed on the open stretches.

Confidence-building obstacle courses, such as the Parachute Regiment's vertiginous 'Trainasium', are more about mental rather than physical training, so might not be considered by the endurance athlete. They can be useful in training for high-altitude environments in which the athlete needs a fearless attitude to heights. The risks of serious injury is very real, however, so check with the course instructors about the safety

Cycling Technique

When cycling, ensure that your leg does not fully straighten on the down push. Your toes should just touch the ground when off the pedals.

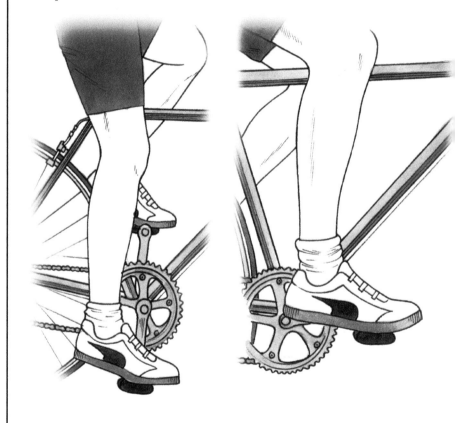

measures in place to reduce the risk of accidents.

Note that the military world does not have the monopoly on ultimate endurance obstacle courses. If you are prepared to travel, you will usually be able to access good civilian courses, including some with fearsome reputations. Of international repute are the Tough Mudder challenges, 16–19km

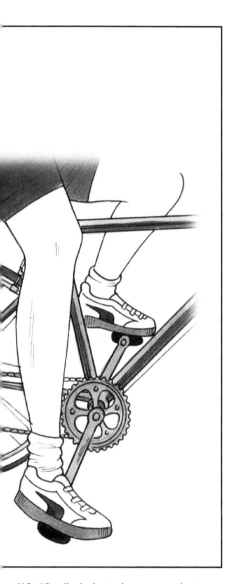

Cycling

Any discussion of extreme fitness would be incomplete without a consideration of cycling. Cycling is both a hugely popular sport in its own right, as well as a good component in cross-training. Like swimming, cycling has the advantage of being relatively kind to the joints, the circular motion of the pedals being gentler on the lower-limb joints than running. But there the gentleness ends, for cycling is a serious endurance sport. The athletes who complete the Tour de France, for example, travel 3200km (2000 miles) in 21 days, surmounting mountain ranges that would challenge a walker, let alone someone on a bike. Such individuals have unsurpassed cardiovascular fitness, as well as leg and core muscles of iron.

Competitive cycling is a diverse sport, with many different sub-categories of event. These include mountain biking, time-trialling, cyclo-cross, track cycling, BMX and cycle speedway. Rather than attempt to unpack the secrets behind each of these, here we will profitably look at the general principles of how to improve cycling speed, whether on rough track or smooth road.

Cycling obviously begins with the purchase of a bike. Invest in a quality machine if you intend to do serious mileage; you want a bike that is both light and strong, and which can be easily configured for your personal body shape.

(10–12 miles) obstacle courses that are both fun and truly exhausting to complete. Undertaking such a course easily ranks alongside marathons in terms of physical achievements.

Road Race

Road racing test
endurance, motor
skills and the ability to
handle a bike safely in
crowded, fast-moving
conditions. Races
often cover difficult
terrain and include
a variety of climbs
and rapid ascents.
Experienced riders
will often ride in the
slipstream of those
in front to ease
energy expenditure.

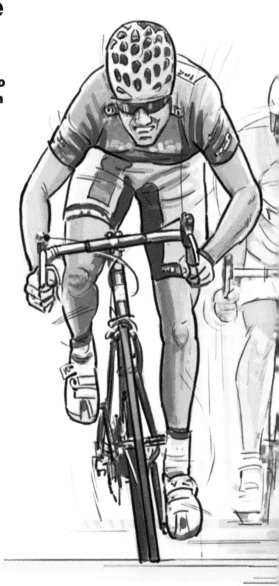

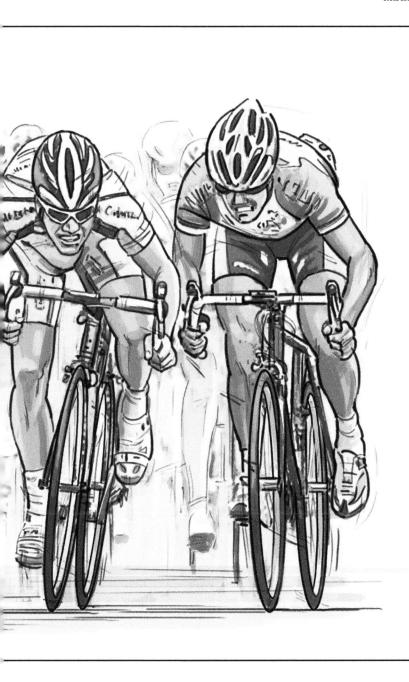

You should have the bike properly adjusted for your height and body shape. This set-up needs to be done accurately, or not only will cycling be an uncomfortable experience, but you will also slow yourself down by increasing wind drag and having an awkward pedalling action. In terms of saddle height, at the bottom of the pedal stroke the leg should nearly be straight, but with a slight bend at the knee of about 25 degrees.

If the angle of bend is more or less than this, then your cycling action will be less efficient (particularly at your leg's maximum extension) and your could be storing up knee problems for later on in life. When the pedals are in their central (or horizontal) position, the knee should be either directly above or just slightly in front of the pedal crank arm.

In terms of the handlebar position, when the hands are gripping the tops of the handlebars (as opposed to the drops, on a racing bike), the back should be at a 45-degree relation to the ground. For road racing, the back should also have a slight upward flex in it to help the spine absorb the inevitable shocks imparted by the road surface. (Don't allow your back to collapse too far forward into an inflexible concave position.) Keep your neck in a neutral position, and look forward rather than down at the road.

Reducing Muscular Pain

It is vital for any sort of endurance cycling that you keep your body as relaxed as possible, otherwise any tension will build up into muscular pain as you rack up the miles. Don't throttle the handlebars – keep the grip gentle, loose but controlled. For a general relaxed position place your hands on the tops of the handlebars or on the brake hoods; the classic road racing position, however, involves gripping the handlebar drops, which pushes the back down further and therefore increases the aerodynamic configuration of the rider. Elbows need to be flexed slightly, the bend providing a shock-absorber effect for the upper body while also giving you more control over cornering. Shoulders are relaxed and never hunched.

Your body position in any cycling sport will obviously change according to the nature of the terrain. When climbing steep inclines, for example, the buttocks should be further back on the saddle and the hands on the tops of the handlebars. This position opens up the chest, aiding the deep respiration required for a difficult climb.

Going downhill, the buttocks are more in the middle of the saddle, with the hands in the drops to maximize speed. Keeping the hands in the drops is also a good tip for fast cornering, as the position lowers the

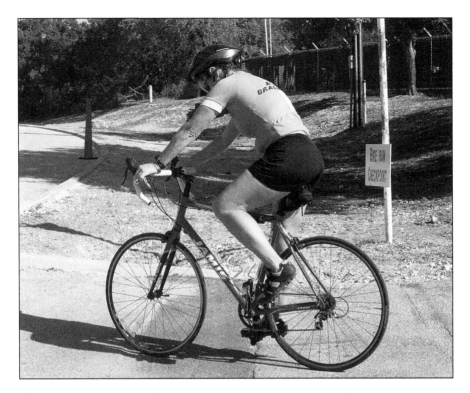

Cycling is an excellent low-impact exercise, useful to give your body a break when you have been working at high-impact resistance training. Note the soft position of the elbows and loose, but firm, grip.

centre of gravity and – combined with the cyclist shifting his body weight slightly into the corner – gives the bike better adhesion to the road.

If your chosen cycle sport involves maintaining speed over long distances, your training should focus on building a fast and smooth pedalling cadence ('cadence' refers simply to the number of revolutions of the pedals per minute). Professional cyclists can aim for a cadence of about 90rpm on long, flat sections, and 70rpm on steep hill climbs. Don't select a gear that is too high for good cadence; instead go for a gear in which you can keep a rapid rhythm flowing smoothly and continually. Apply power through the entire cycle of the pedal, not just on the downward thrust.

You can improve you pedal cadence through a variety of speed drills. A useful exercise is to cycle at a fast rate of about 90–100rpm in an easy gear for five minutes, then switch back to your normal gearing for ten minutes, repeating the process throughout the ride. Using interval training such as this, you will find that your legs eventually adjust to both higher gearing and faster cadence, producing much better race times. When doing speed pedalling, however, make sure that you go as fast as you can without bouncing in the saddle.

Stop immediately if you begin to experience any knee pain.

Off-road Cycling
Mountain biking has a range of different concerns to road/track racing, especially in terms of safe manoeuvring. When descending, for example, you must control your speed sufficiently to manage all corners; use your front and back brakes together to keep your momentum manageable.

U.S. Army Tip – Progression and Recovery

Other important principles for avoiding injury are progression and recovery. Programs that try to do too much too soon invite problems. The day after a 'hard' training day, if soldiers are working the same muscle groups and/or fitness components, they should work them at a reduced intensity to minimize stress and permit recovery. The best technique is to train alternate muscle groups and/or fitness components on different days. For example, if the Monday–Wednesday–Friday (M-W-F) training objective is CR fitness, soldiers can do ability group running at THR with some light calisthenics and stretching. If the Tuesday–Thursday (T-Th) objective is muscular endurance and strength, soldiers can benefit from doing partner-resisted exercises followed by a slow run. To ensure balance and regularity in the program, the next week should have muscle endurance and strength development on M-W-F and training for CR endurance on T-Th. Such a program has variety, develops all the fitness components and follows the seven principles of exercise while, at the same time, it minimizes injuries caused by overuse.

– U.S. Army, FM 21-20, 8-1

Mountain Biking

Mountain biking not only builds leg strength, the constant adjustments in balance develop the core muscles.

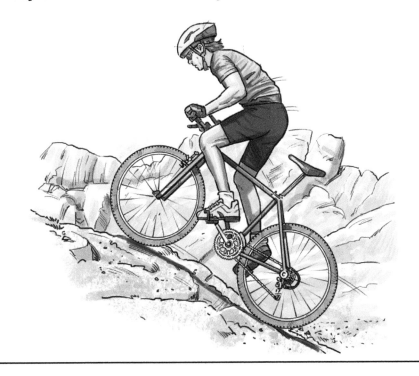

When attacking a hill, don't just automatically drop down to the lowest gear and hit the hill fast. Instead, shift your weight back on the saddle and choose a gear just low enough so that you don't have to stand on the pedals. Keep your eyes forward and choose you line around corners and obstacles intelligently. For uphill switchbacks, place your wheel on the outer edge of the corner until you straighten across the track in the last quarter of the turn, and select a gear low enough to maintain a powerful cadence throughout the manoeuvre. Downhill switchbacks require that you shave off speed through braking before you enter the corner. Follow the same sort of line as the uphill switchback,

Regaining the Advantage

In floor grappling, get your arms and legs into bent defensive positions as soon as you can. Not only will this protect you from further assault, but it might be your only chance to strike back and regain the advantage.

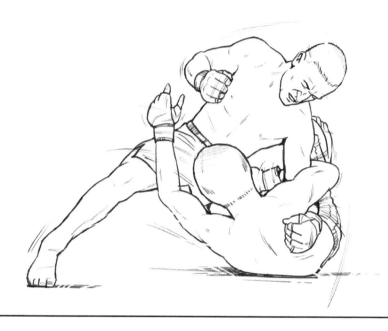

but keep your weight back to reduce skidding. Lean your body to the inside of the turn while pushing your lower weight (through your legs) to the outside; this posture will help keep your front wheel on the ground and give you better control around the line of the turn.

You can support your efficiency as a cyclist with cross-training. Circuits, running, swimming and weight training are all good options, as they will help you build up your stamina levels across the board.

Martial Arts

The martial arts, in which we include boxing, are superb sports to practice in themselves, or to add to a cross-training programme. Anyone who has attempted a single minute of full-power workout on a punch bag

Roundhouse Kick

Although this soldier can kick to head height, you should only practice kicks within the limits of your flexibility, thereby avoiding groin and hamstring injuries.

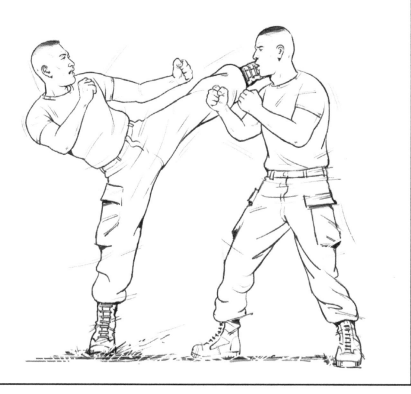

will soon realize that the fitness levels of professional boxers are near superhuman levels, especially as they have to cope with the additional exhaustion of coping with powerful blows. Martial arts such as karate, taekwondo, judo and ju-jitsu are exceptional for producing flexibility and explosive anaerobic fitness; many of the better martial arts classes will also incorporate aerobic endurance training to ensure the participants have no chinks in their physical armour. Furthermore, martial

Sparring

The goal of military sparring is not typically a knockout or win, but to improve stamina and agility while practising defending, taking and inflicting blows.

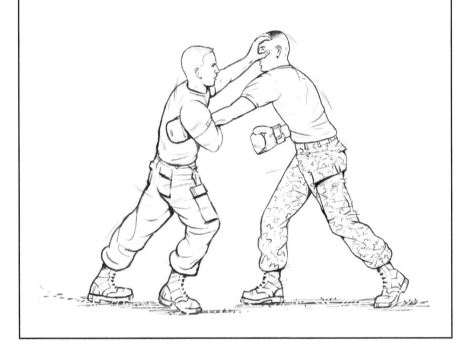

arts obviously train the individual in the skills of self-defence, a worthy pursuit in its own right.

Unarmed combat naturally has a central place in military training. While some special forces have their own bespoke varieties of martial art – such as the Israeli krav maga – most opt for a practical combat training that mixes punching, kicking, choking, locking and throwing

techniques, rather like ju-jitsu. Boxing is often added to provide a bit of amateur aggression testing. In the British Parachute Regiment, for example, recruits undergo the infamous 'milling' test, where two recruits box each other ferociously for a solid minute, the instructors looking for demonstrations of guts and spirit, rather than any form of refined technique.

Grappling

An excellent workout, grappling consists of techniques and counters designed to takedown, throw or pin your opponent in a submission hold.

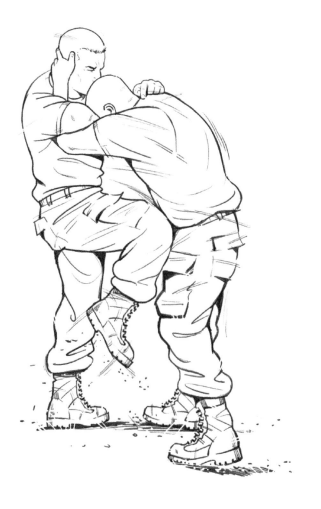

Using Pads

Aim to strike the centre of the pad with the correct part of your hand, foot, elbow or knee. Have your training partner alter the pad presentations constantly, forcing you to adjust your techniques.

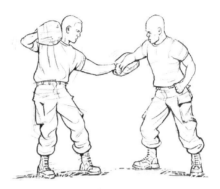

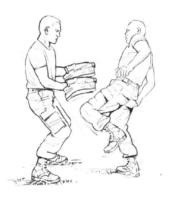

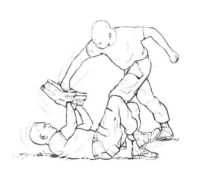

Traditional martial arts often focus on one or two aspects of this spectrum nearly exclusively. Taekwondo and karate, for example, give privilege to kicking and straight-arm punching techniques, while judo emphasises holds and grappling. Practised with commitment, all martial arts will provide good fitness training. For cross-training to support endurance sports, however, there are a handful of techniques that are particularly useful.

Building Stamina

Striking punchbags or focus mitts is a concentrated way of building both aerobic and anaerobic stamina. The constant impacts quickly drain your strength and stretch your cardiovascular limits, while also strengthening the core, back, shoulder and arm muscles. Before you start striking hard, ensure that you get some training in correct punching technique. Your jabs and crosses need to be pushed out straight, with the elbow kept behind the punch and not allowed to swing outwards. (Soldiers are also taught that letting your elbow swing out makes it easier for your opponent to see the punch coming and dodge it.) If you are not wearing boxing gloves or similar hand protection (such protection is advised if you

U.S. Army Tip – Using Foam Pads

Foam pads are highly recommended to enhance training. The pads allow full-forced strikes by soldiers and protect their training partners. The pads enable soldiers to feel the effectiveness of striking techniques and to develop power in their striking. Instructors should encourage spirited aggressiveness. Pads can be tackle dummy pads or martial arts striking pads. The use of pads is especially recommended for knee-strike practice drills, kicking drills and three-foot-stick striking drills. The pad is ideally placed on the outside of the training partner's thigh, protecting the common peroneal nerve. Pads can also be held against the forearms in front of the head and face to allow practice knee/elbow strikes to this area.

– U.S. Army, FM 21-150, *Combatives*, 2-27

Kick Pads

When delivering any blow to a pad, fix your eyes on the intended impact point. Retain control of your balance at all times, and recover your guard stance smoothly and quickly.

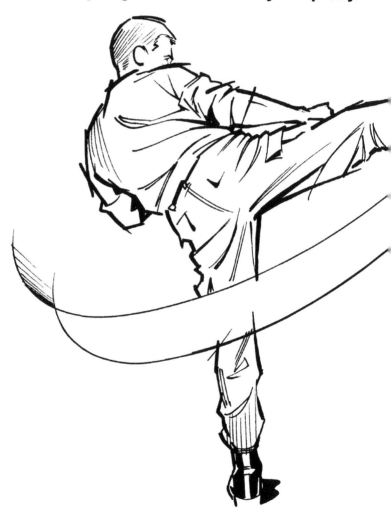

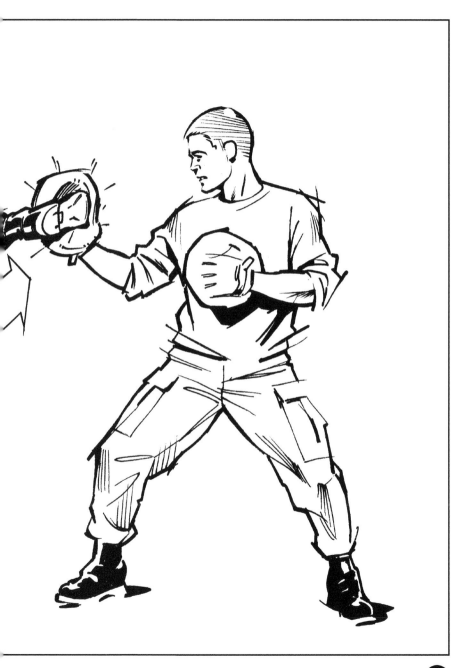

Using a Kick Bag

Kick bags are useful in that they provide a realistic gauge of the power of your kick. Lean you body weight into the blow for max effect.

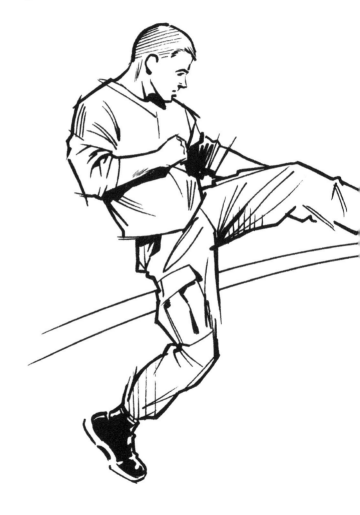

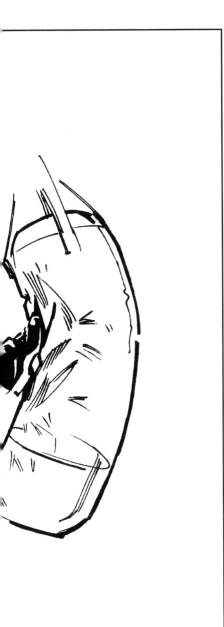

are not properly trained), make sure that the back of your hand is flat in line with the back of the forearm, and that the impact point is the two large knuckles at the top of the fist. The fist itself should be made tightly, with the fingers pulled back hard into the palm and the thumb tucked away safely on the outside (never gripped within the fingers).

Practise throwing fast, hard combinations at the pad, keeping light on your toes and with the left foot forward (if you are right-handed), your body balanced at all times. When you throw the punch, keep your arm as relaxed as possible for most of the flight; a relaxed muscle is a fast muscle. Then as you strike the pad, tense your body from your toes to your shoulders, to give the punch a solid base and avoid having the weight of the punch bag force you backwards. This repeated relax/tense pattern is superb conditioning for your core muscles, which – along with the huge amount of abdominal exercises they do – helps explain why boxers usually have such exceptional definition in their stomach muscles.

When practising kicking techniques, these should be performed within the limits of your flexibility to avoid sudden strains to the groin, hamstrings or other lower-body muscles. Techniques such as roundhouse kicks or spinning kicks need special attention to technique. For example, avoid performing a

U.S. Army Tip – Buddy-assisted Groin (Butterfly) Stretch

a. Position: Sit on ground with the soles of your feet together, close to the torso. Hold ankles with hands. Have your buddy kneel behind you with his hands on your knees.

b. Action: Your buddy places his hands on top of your thighs at the knees. His weight is supported by your shoulders while little weight is placed on the thighs. Then, your buddy increases downward pressure on your thighs until stretch is felt. Hold for 20 seconds, then alternate positions.

roundhouse kick with the supporting foot pointing forward, as this will subject the lower back to high levels of torsion and run the risk of muscle strain. Instead, in the kick's final position the supporting foot should be roughly at the seven o'clock position relative to the impact point, the side of the body fully aligned with the extension of the kick. The same applies to any side-thrust kick.

Stretching and flexibility training are typically integral to the martial arts, so your ability to kick higher will come gradually. Some martial arts classes can perform very aggressive stretching exercises using partners to apply extra pressure to the limbs. This is fine as long as you dictate the limit of the stretch at all times. As always, if you have any pain during the stretch, stop immediately.

Triathlons

The acid test of cross-training is the triathlon event. As the introduction to this chapter indicated, triathlons stretch the all-round fitness levels of an athlete in ways that few other sports can do. The popularity of triathlons is also increasing at impressive levels (more than 30 per cent in the United States between 2003 and 2008).

Being a three-sport activity, your training for a triathlon obviously needs to incorporate all three elements. This can be a challenge in itself in terms of finding the time to devote training to each aspect equally. Most important is that you work on developing excellent technique in all three disciplines, as energy conservation is critical to performing a good triathlon. Your training week

A Winning Mentality

Add continuous challenges to your training, such as races, gradings or triathlons, to instil motivation.

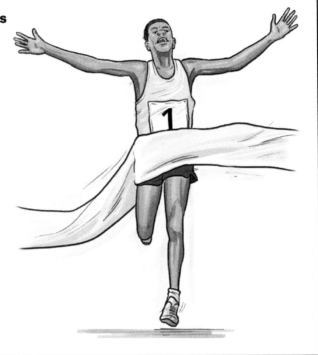

should incorporate all the sports individually, but also at least a day when you combine all three. These days are especially important as they give you the opportunity to practice the transitions between each activity. Typically, leg muscles feel weak when going from, for example, swimming to running, and if you are not used to this sensation you could experience a significant drop in your available energy levels. In all three disciplines, vary the intensity and pace of your routines to get used to applying power when required. During the race itself you can treat the first half much like a marathon, holding back your energy so that you can apply it at the right time during the later stages, such as when you are sprinting for the finish.

Triathlons, like any endurance sport, can bring a tremendous sense of satisfaction. If you are a triathlon novice, start small and work your way up through bigger events.

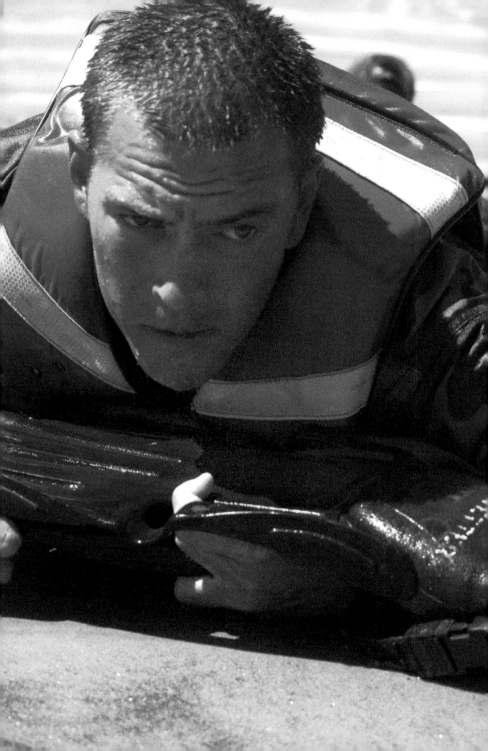

In the 1980s and 1990s, psychologists began to take a keen interest in a relatively new field of their profession. Responding to a prevailing attitude among sports trainers that success was more mental than physical, they began to implement tests to see whether that assertion was indeed true and whether some form of purely mental training could enhance physical action. They implemented a large number of experiments (and are still doing so today), some focusing just on the relationship between mental training and general motor skills and others looking at the mind and its connection to sporting performance. The principal focus of the studies was visualization – the practice of vividly imaging, in a controlled and systematic way, performing an action in a perfect style – and its correlation with improvements in the skills visualized.

The results that steadily emerged were undeniable. Physical practice at a sport remained, and remains, key – you cannot simply imagine your way to excellence in a sport without also putting in the hours of practice. However, what did become clear was that those athletes who invested in visualization or similar forms of

....

Opposite: The ability to carry on when others might fail is a defining feature of special forces personnel.

7

The theme of mental preparation is one that has run throughout this book. Very high levels of physical fitness will take you so far in performing extreme fitness challenges, but mental focus and preparation will take you the rest of the way.

Mental Preparation

Fatigue and Support

Know your own limits – accepting assistance is not necessarily a sign of weakness if it helps prevent injury.

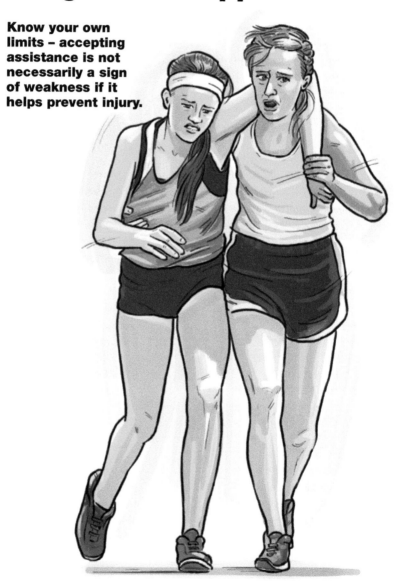

mental training, generally experienced real-world improvements in their sporting achievements. The message is clear – to excel at any sport you should train your mind as well as your body. The military has always delved, to some degree, into mental training, whether it knew it or not. The arduous training, discipline, rituals, battlefield camaraderie, uniforms, decorations (unit and individual), shared ordeals, remembrance days and unit pride (often inculcated through its history) work towards instilling the personal motivation and group thinking that lead to a cohesive and effective force. As with the study of sports psychology, the military has also now professionalized its approach to mental training, psychologists becoming more central to constructing training programmes and maintaining the soldier's long-term welfare. In this chapter, we will bring together both military and sports psychology, and see how they can help athletes attain peak performance in the most demanding of sports.

Shaping the Individual

During the recruitment and selection phases of military training, the primary goal of the instructors is nearly universal. The training is intended to take the raw material of a young man (or woman), undo any bad habits he has developed in civilian life (and get rid of him if he doesn't shape up), foster the good habits and rebuild him in the military's image of an effective warrior. Not everyone responds to this treatment. Modern recruiters and instructors often complain that modern living tends to breed individuals used to comfort and emotional indulgence. Around 50 years ago, most people (certainly enlisted men) entering the armed forces would have been used to a certain degree of physical hardship. Those brought up in tough physical circumstances become adept at the mental habits of self-denial and emotional resilience, traits that have an obvious relevance for military units. Today, TV, centrally heated/air-conditioned homes, a high level of social services provision, plentiful food, low levels of physical activity (partly the product of increased use of video games) and a more protection-focused environment means that recruits tend to arrive at boot camp somewhat 'softer' than previous generations.

In 2010, press reports revealed that the U.S. Army frequently had to modify its training programmes significantly to accommodate this new generation, reducing the initial intensity of the physical training and building it up more slowly, with less verbal and emotional aggression from the instructors. Captain Scott Sewell, an army trainer, told the Associated Press that: 'Most of these soldiers have never been in a fistfight or any

Paralympics

**Military training techniques can apply
to anyone with the determination to win.
The Paralympics enables those with a
range of disabilities, including amputees
and the wheelchair-bound, to compete at
world-class levels.**

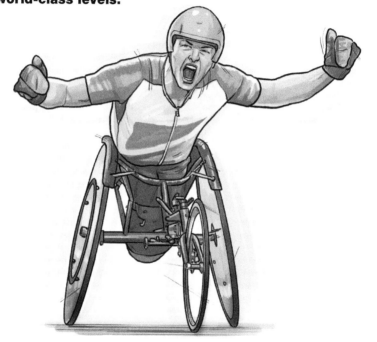

kind of a physical confrontation. They are stunned when they get smacked in the face. We are trying to get them to act, to think like warriors.'

The 'think like warriors' goal is crucial to the armed forces. The military is not interested in people who just go through the motions, those who simply do enough to stay the course. Instead they want people who are warriors to the very core, individuals who are utterly motivated by their own professionalism and their desire to complete any given mission. So how is this attitude instilled? The conventional routes are as follows:

Comradeship

Professional armies frequently use a buddy system, meaning that soldiers are paired for mutual support. A close friend can act as your 'buddy' during extreme fitness training.

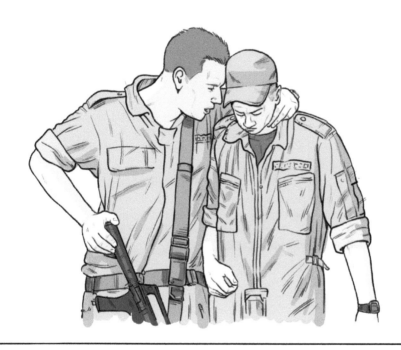

- **Discipline** – the soldier is trained to follow orders and repeatedly perform onerous tasks to high standards. The process of repetition instils discipline as a habit, rather than just an occasional practice. (According to recent psychological investigations, habits are established after about 28 days of continual reinforcement of the target behaviour.)

- **Cultivated aggression** – through combat and (often brutal) unarmed combat training, the soldier learns to channel aggression, at the same time overriding fear and learning to cope with the adrenaline of physical danger and confrontation.

- **Battle inoculation** – this distinctive phrase refers to a more modern trend in military training, in which ultra-realistic training conditions are used to familiarize the soldier with the mental and physical sensations of combat, making him less likely to freeze or panic in actual life-threatening situations.

- **Pride** – instructors and officers should imbue the soldiers with a deep-felt sense of unit pride, imparted through meaningful rituals, unit history, a competitive spirit, uniforms and insignia and any other inspirational tools. The soldier should feel that he belongs to something bigger than himself.

- **Comradeship** – military units are intense social groups, with soldiers often stating that the bonds they form with their unit members have a greater emotional strength than many family ties. Good soldiers strive to do their best because they have an intense fear of letting their comrades and unit down.

In addition to the above, the U.S. Army in particular has introduced extensive new systems of mental training. Since 2009, and in an effort to reduce the number of post-traumatic stress disorder (PTSD) victims returning from combat theatres, the army has implemented the Comprehensive Soldier and Family Fitness Program (CSFFP). This programme in turn builds upon the Total Force Fitness (TFF) initiative introduced two years previously, described as 'a framework for building and maintaining health, readiness and performance in the Department of Defence. It views health, wellness and resilience as a holistic concept where optimal performance requires a connection between mind, body, spirit and family/social relationships' (hprc-online.org/total-force-fitness). The concept of 'resilience' is key to both the CSFFP and TFF, being a state of mind capable of enduring hard circumstances without experiencing mental damage.

The main training objectives of the soldier component of CSFFP are:

• Building confidence – develop effective thinking skills to create energy, optimism and enthusiasm and help manage internal obstacles that hinder performance excellence.

• Attention control – employ methods to take control of your attention, improve your ability to attend fully and concentrate amidst distractions.

• Energy management – use self-regulation skills to effectively

Controlled Aggression

Channeling your aggression
so that it works for you, not
against you, is essential
for success in the military.
Imagine your adrenaline is
like a tap, which you can
turn on and off as required.

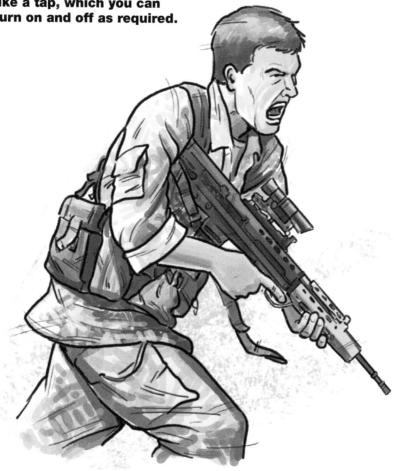

modulate and restore energy in order to thrive under pressure.
• *Goal setting – develop a concrete, step-by-step plan for achieving a personally meaningful goal and maintaining the motivation necessary to be successful.*
• *Integrating imagery – mentally rehearse successful performances to program the mind and body to perform automatically and without hesitation.*
– Source: csf2.army.mil/ performance-enhancement.html

The ultimate goal of mastering each of these stages is known as 'mental strength for life'. Looking at the list we can immediately see the value of these principles for those who participate in extreme fitness activities. The components are essentially about confidence and focus, developing a blend of self-belief and a powerful focus on goals. Taking these principles as foundations, we are now going to explore the mental techniques for improving your athletic output. In doing so we will draw continually on the expertise of the military, who every year elicit peak performance from thousands of raw recruits.

Mental Preparation

Mental preparation requires a degree of organization to be effective. At its most basic, this means developing a positive attitude to problems as a *habit*, something deeply ingrained into your mental fabric. Producing a 'can do' attitude is something that is central to the military ethos, and if practised often enough will form a bedrock for tackling extreme fitness challenges.

Faced with the frequent boredoms and frustrations of daily life, it is all too easy to fall into a more despondent mindset, with the consequent effects in missed training sessions and failure to achieve one's goals. Therefore the principles of mental fitness outlined below need frequent and conscious repetition if they are to be of any value. Your character, like your body, behaves very much like a muscle – that which you do frequently becomes stronger, and that which you do infrequently grows weaker. This applies to bad habits as well as good, and is a root explanation for human maladies such as serious addictions. It pays, therefore, to do an audit of all your daily habits, the behaviours (internal or external) that you do frequently. Be honest here, and see how those behaviours contribute towards your fitness goals. For example, you might have fallen into a bad habit of

Opposite: The military selection process is design to weed out those who can't exhibit mental and physical self-discipline.

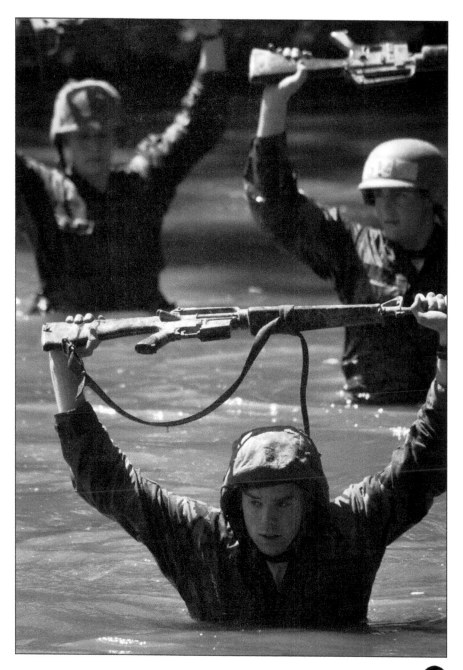

Reminders of Home

Carrying reminders of home and family when far away can help alleviate negativity and remind you what you are working towards.

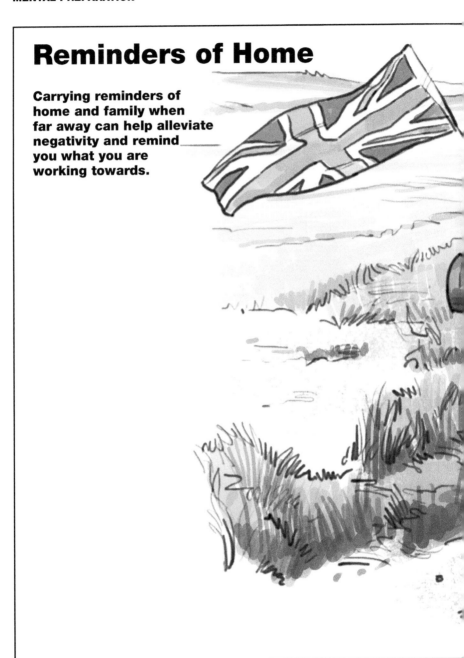

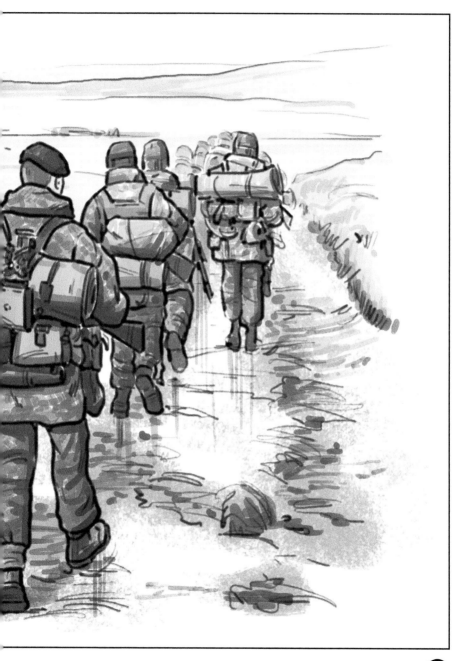

Pole Vault

Pole vaulting requires speed, agility and core strength, as well as complete mental focus on the bar towering above you. Any indecision or mental wavering can result in a dangerous accident.

missing breakfast, but then binging on sweets or biscuits midmorning to restore your energy levels. You might have slipped into the habit of mentally berating yourself every time you run poorly, and then dropping the next few training sessions in frustration (you might be missing an obvious issue, like building rest days into your training programme).

Military units, at least the good ones, have an extremely well developed culture of self-criticism, in which they take apart their processes and performance with an often brutal honesty. Having identified the problems, they then set about remedying them with concrete and efficient steps. As an endurance athlete, you need a similarly robust and inquisitive approach to your own problems. The following processes will help you to ensure that mental and physical development go hand in hand.

Define Your Goals

This piece of sounds obvious, but too often goals are defined in woolly or weak terms that do not generate enough internal motivation. The key is to make your objective sharp. Thus instead of saying: 'My goal is to perform a major endurance run', it is far better to define your goal as something like: 'My goal is to run the <venue> marathon on <date> in <time>'. Defining the objective in sharp and concrete terms means

that all your efforts now have a clear direction of energy. In military speak, regard your objective as your *mission*, a term that carries with it a rounder sense of obligation and focus. As the U.S. Marine manual *Warfighting* explains regarding military operations: 'The first requirement is to establish what we want to accomplish, why and how. Without a clearly identified concept and intent, the necessary unity of effort is inconceivable' (USMC, *Warfighting*, p.82). Also avoid including negative objectives in your mission, as they can remind you of your failures, with a knock-on demotivation. So avoid goals such as 'I want to stop eating all the unhealthy food I seem to crave', say 'I will eat a wholesome and nutritious diet and be in control of everything I eat.' Note the imperative sense of 'I will…' – it can help to phrase you goal in terms that imply certain achievement, so you can start to feel the energy provided by expectation.

Break Down the Whole

Once you have established your goal, make sure that you don't allow it to intimidate you with its scale. Most accomplishments in life are made through small, incremental steps towards the objective, not immediate and dramatic leaps. Therefore, break down your large goal into manageable chunks and direct your focus on accomplishing the sub-goals one at a time. Also, be adaptable – if

Milling

The British Parachute Regiment uses milling as a means of controlled aggression and preparation for live combat. Technique is not important – total commitment and ferocity are the key factors.

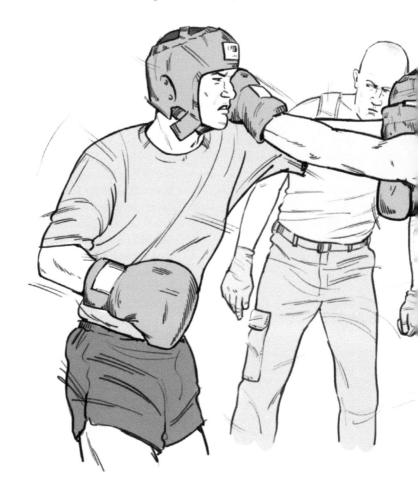

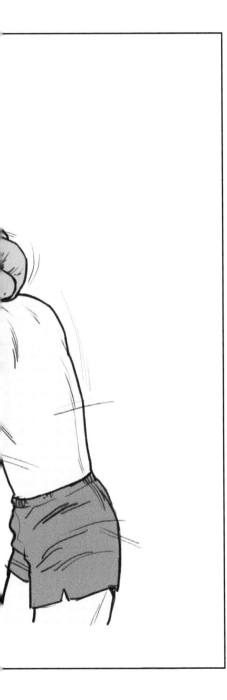

something really isn't working for you, change your training method until you get back on track.

The U.S. Marine Corps operate what some analysts have called a '70 per cent solution'. Here the overall plan has at least a 70 per cent chance of working in its unmodified state. A 100 per cent certain plan is usually not sought, because life rarely pans out as planned, and rigid thinking can prevent you being adaptable to circumstances as they arise. Instead, work step by step towards your objective, and shift tactics as necessary. In other words, don't change you end goal, but do change the means by which you get there.

Visualize

Special Forces military training has seriously embraced the relevance of visualization as part of its modern training programme. Elite units such as the U.S. Navy SEALs and U.S. Army Special Forces have all invested research and study into the benefits of visualization training as part of what they variously call 'Emergency Conditioning' (EC) or 'battle inoculation'.

In basic outline, the essence of visualization techniques is that the individual can condition himself better to achieve goals or survive adversity by vividly imaging his actions within the challenging scenarios. If a situation is mentally rehearsed with enough clarity and realism, that mental image then enters the mental files of a person's experience. Hence when the individual encounters that situation for real, they are more likely to adopt the positive responses they practised under the controlled conditions of visualization.

In terms of visualization for extreme fitness training, there are two basic types: 1. Pre-event visualization; 2. In-event visualization. Pre-event visualization involves you mentally rehearsing exactly how you want to perform during a fitness challenge. To do this efficiently, lie or sit in a quiet place with your eyes closed, and for at least five minutes just focus on the slow rise and fall of your own breathing, relaxing deeper with every exhalation. If unwanted thoughts enter your mind, just let them pass through without emotion or reflection, like images in a movie you aren't really watching. Once you are mentally and physically relaxed, picture the event you want to visualize.

The key to making this process effective is to recreate the situation in great detail and authenticity. If you are imagining a mountain run, for example, 'see' the colour of the grass and rocks around you, and the sky above you; 'hear' the noise of your shoes hitting the surface, and your breathing; 'feel' the aches in your muscles or the sweat trickling down the side of your face. Basically add as much detail as possible, and then within that scenario picture yourself at peak performance. Imagine yourself powering with confidence and stamina up the steepest parts of the course, passing other competitors as you go. Imagine your energy levels constant and strong, your spirits high. Once you have played out the scenario for as long as you feel necessary, bring yourself out of your relaxed state by counting from one to five, feeling more wakeful as you ascend the numbers.

This type of visualization works essentially as a form of mental programming, providing your brain with a model of peak performance that will, hopefully, replay itself in actuality when you later tackle the challenge. You can also use visualization techniques during an event itself to help you keep pushing through mental and physical barriers. Here you can be truly creative.

For example, when I am struggling up a mountainside, I imagine that I have a big motorbike engine set inside my chest, throbbing powerfully and providing motive force directly to my legs. I literally turn my right hand, revving the 'throttle' and imagine that the engine is driving me effortlessly up the hill. My wife (also a runner) imagines crowds of people either side of her, cheering her on to greatness. Develop your own personal range of mental aids, based on things that inspire you directly, and utilize them when you most need them.

Visualization Techniques

While its benefits might seem unrealistic at first, visualization can have a positive and powerful effect in helping you achieve your goals.

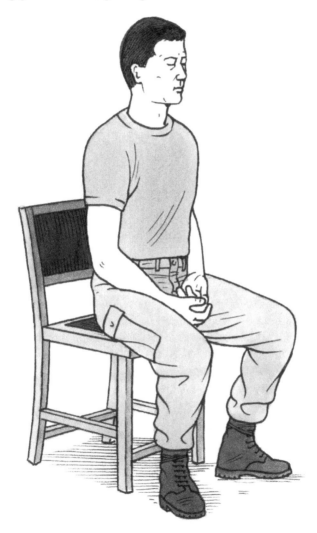

Mental Anaesthesia

Visualization has a proven role in pain relief, including for managing pain in endurance sports. One particular technique is known as 'mental anaesthesia'. To understand this, imagine that a pain-killing injection is being applied directly to the site of the pain. The pain dissolves under the influence of the injection; it can sometimes help to imagine a beautiful, warm yellow liquid spreading around and absorbing the pain. Another technique is to imagine that you have a tap that controls the flow of sensation from the pain to your brain. When the pain gets too much, simply imagine closing the tap, stopping the flow of pain and isolating it. Play around with similar techniques until you find one that works for you.

Meditate

Meditation might sound to many as if it belongs in the realms of Eastern mysticism, but the military community is slowly waking up to its potential as a tool to molding effective warriors. In fact, controlled experiments in meditation were conducted within a small group of U.S. Special Forces soldiers in the mid 1980s, led by Vietnam veteran and psychologist Richard Strozzi-Heckler. Strozzi-Heckler implemented a variety of mental training practices, but regular daily meditation seemed to have particular benefit. After weeks of meditating, the soldiers showed definite improvements not only with coping mechanisms while under stress, but also cognitive function and sensory awareness.

Although investigation into the benefits of meditation then trailed off in the military over subsequent decades, it has come back in recent times. At the time of writing (2013), the U.S. Marine Corps is awaiting the results of a pilot programme into the effects of 'mindfulness meditation' on soldiers as a way to improve combat performance and reduce incidents of PTSD.

Scientific research into meditation has revealed an amazing host of psychological and physiological benefits, which include:

- Better stress control and emotional balance
- Improved memory and reasoning
- Improved immune system function

Managing Stress

Stress causes hormones to flood your nervous system. The resulting physical symptoms include a racing pulse and quick, shallow breaths. Act as soon as the effects manifest themselves, taking charge of your body posture and inner voice.

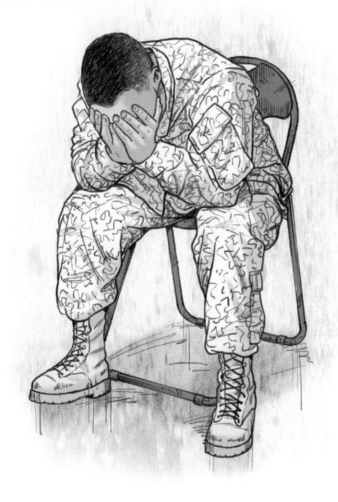

Meditation

The concentrated focus on breathing, or on whatever word or mantra works for you, has long been proven to help clear the mind following stressful situations and can enable you stay in control during major sporting challenges.

- Better digestion (including relief from irritable bowel syndrome)
- Increased levels of fertility
- Lower blood pressure
- Lower incidents of arthritis and other inflammatory conditions

For these physical reasons alone, it is obvious that any endurance athlete would find meditation to be time well spent. Furthermore, although athletes often find intense satisfaction from doing their sport, they still experience the pressure of racing and the strains of daily training, to which they can add the general frustrations of everyday life. If they go into a race a ball of anxiety, the tension will affect muscular strength, flexibility and endurance – meditation can be a switch to turn off such anxiety. Recent studies among U.S. Navy SEALs, U.S. Army Rangers and other Special Forces show that meditation results in more activity in the brain's pre-frontal cortex, which gives the individual a calmer perspective on stressful events and reduces the activity in the amygdala, the brain's fight-or-flight centre.

Mindfulness Meditation

Mindfulness meditation is simple to perform, but requires some discipline. The basic technique begins when you find somewhere quiet where you won't be disturbed. Sit or lie in a comfortable position, close your eyes, then focus your attention on nothing but the smooth rise and fall of your breath, breathing in deeply through your nose and releasing the breath from your mouth. Imagine that you are *staring* mentally at the breath, aware of everything from the noise it makes to the rise and fall of your chest. With each exhalation, consciously relax your muscles as if they were butter softening under a gentle, warm sun. Instead of concentrating on the breath, you might choose a different focus, such as the vocalization 'Om', or a mantra – a simple, gentle word repeated calmly in the mind. Whatever the case, you need a calming and regularly repeated point of focus for your mind.

As you maintain this action, you will find that your brain can fight back. Images and thoughts will crowd into the vacuum, including your anxieties, frustrations and fears. How you react is critical. Don't dwell on the thoughts, but instead just see them without emotion and let them pass like images on a movie screen, returning your focus to your breathing. This process trains your mind to respond reflectively and calmly to your stressors.

If you have never practised meditation you might be surprised at how hard it is. After a couple of minutes you will likely struggle to maintain focus on your breathing, instead getting distracted by your

Seeking Advice

True mental toughness is being able to recognize and admit that you need help. If the solutions outlined in this chapter do not help, try talking issues through with a friend, doctor or professional.

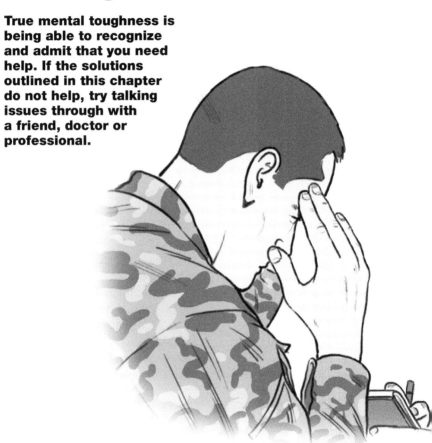

worries, and feeling restless. Yet you should persist, building up your meditative muscle from just a few minutes to at least 15 minutes. Then you will begin to experience the benefits outlined above, and onwards for the rest of your life.

Meditate frequently in the run-up to a big race, or during an intense training period, and you will find yourself more able to cope with pressures, more accepting of the occasional off day and more physically relaxed as your train.

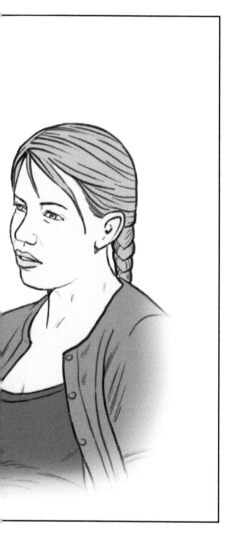

states, revealed courtesy of modern psychological research.

One key trait you can develop to control your mental state is what Richard Wiseman, Professor of the Public Understanding of Psychology at the University of Hertfordshire, U.K., calls the 'as if' principle. (See his publication *Rip It Up: The Radically New Approach to Changing Your Life.*) Research has revealed that the way we behave physically has more of an effect on our emotions than the way we think. So instead of our emotions shaping our physical expression, it works rather more in the opposite direction. Think of it this way. When you are depressed, you adopt the physical expressions of depression: shallow breathing, folded-up body posture, head down, eyes unfocused, frowning facial expression. If you physically force your body into the opposite posture – chin up, arms and legs unfolded, standing up straight with chest out, breathing deeply and slowly, a smile on your face and a raised brow – it is actually quite difficult to feel depressed. Your body is sending signals to your brain about what mental state you are in. Hold this posture for long enough, even if you don't initially feel it is doing any good, and after a while you will physically reshape your mental state.

The 'as if' principle has great potential for extreme fitness.

Control What Can Be Controlled
Emotional states are fluid and unpredictable qualities, and trying to control them by willpower alone can have frustrated outcomes. Fortunately for the athelete, there are some easier routes to modifying our mental

Brain Training

Taking up an activity such as learning a new instrument, language or skill, is a great way to train under-utilised areas of your brain, as well as being relaxing and enjoyable.

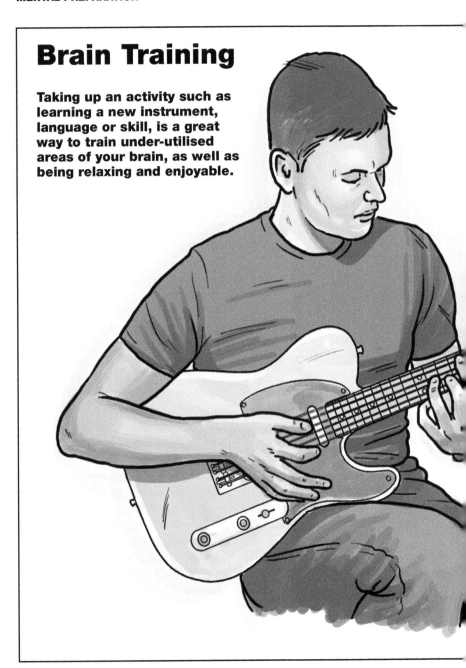

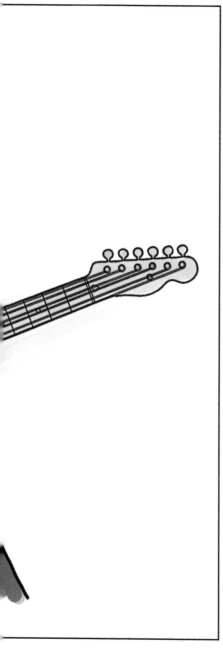

Adopting the physical expressions of confidence and determination will help you to feel that way internally. You can also apply this principle to your internal dialogue. Don't allow negative language to dominate, but instead express your thoughts with confidence and purpose.

Dissociation

One of the benefits of the internet is that many ex-Special Forces soldiers have joined forums and message boards in which they post their reflections on life in the military elite, and how they survived the punishing training regime. The author has spent much time studying these forums, and one particular mental technique emerges – what psychologists would call 'dissociation'. In this mental state, the individual mentally disconnects his emotions from the outer world, while still remaining committed to fulfilling his tasks as effectively as possible. Thus we see many ex-U.S. Navy SEALs talking about surviving 'Hell Week' by simply putting their brains into 'neutral', almost letting their bodies perform the physical challenges while their emotions remained elsewhere. The attitude is that they recognize the pain their bodies are going through, but don't invest that situation with emotional content.

Dissociation is a central building block of resilience. During this state, it is almost as if you are watching

Post-traumatic Stress Disorder

Prolonged exposure to stress or traumatic events is common for serving military personnel. The U.S. Army diagnosed more than 75,000 cases of PTSD between 2000 and 2011.

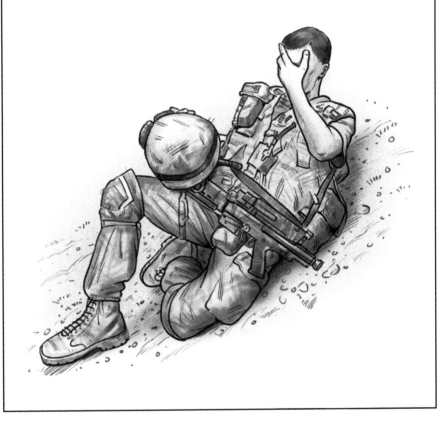

yourself go through hell, but the observer part of you doesn't care. Using the meditative techniques described earlier can also help you improve your skills in dissociation. Obviously, don't dissociate yourself so much from serious issues that you end up ignoring their reality. Any mental technique should enhance your performance, not put you in harm's way.

Relax

Don't forget the importance of relaxation. When you are in the midst of a punishing training schedule, give your mind as well as your body a rest by socializing and investing in fun. Go out, dance, watch movies, walk the dog – anything to help you unwind. Spend time with people you like and who make you laugh. Humour is for my money one of the greatest coping mechanisms there is, which is why military trainers watch candidates closely for their use of humour during training. Those without a good sense of humour under adversity are likely to prove a drain on unit morale, while those who can find the funny side will have a positive influence on all those around them.

Toughen Up

'Toughen up' is not the most nuanced piece of mental advice, but it still has resonance and value. By constantly putting yourself through endurance challenges, you will automatically develop a high degree of mental toughness – you wouldn't be able to continue doing the sport if you didn't. If you feel you need to develop more in the way of 'grit', try the following technique. For a period of 28 days, never complain to anyone about anything (you can, of course,

talk about resolving problems, but do this in a functional way). In other words, don't moan just for the sake of it. If and when you catch yourself doing it, stop immediately and let the desire pass away. You can eventually internalize this process so you don't even moan to yourself, producing a mental hardening that will serve you well during the trials of an extreme fitness event.

Realism

While I have nothing to retract from the statements about mental preparation above, you also have to be realistic about your capabilities. Extreme fitness challenges are often by their nature physically exhausting or even dangerous, and should only be attempted if diligent preparation has made you ready to take them on. Never simply think you can perform heroic endurance feats just on the basis of willpower alone.

An expression commonly used in both military and fitness training is 'Pain is weakness leaving the body.' It is a phrase I find deeply irritating. I understand the sentiment, but there is also the fact that pain, in some forms, can be a justifiable message that something is going terribly wrong. Every year around the world, people die in endurance events because they push their bodies further and harder than their capabilities. Such behaviour is a sad and futile waste of life. I do believe that you should

Pride and Honour

Fulfilling ones goals can give a huge sense of pride. When you achieve a goal, reinforce the sense of achievement through simple rituals or celebrations.

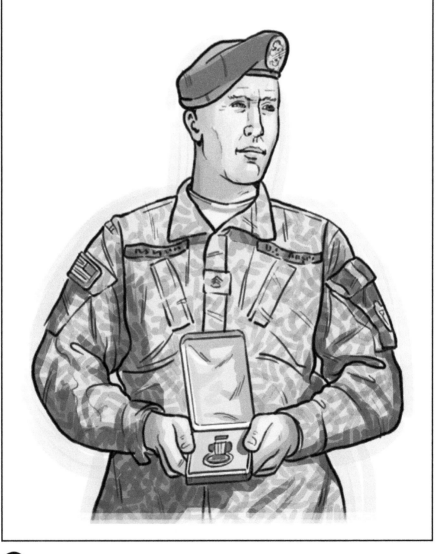

Leadership

**Being able to remain
in control and make
informed decisions
when surrounded
by fear and chaos
is the mark of a
true military leader.
In athletic events,
leadership of yourself
may well be the
greatest challenge.**

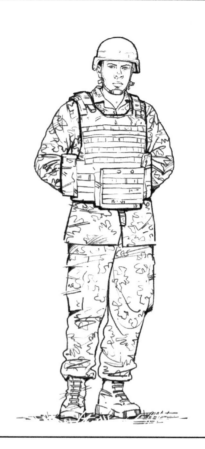

drive yourself to the limit, using all the mental and physical tools at your disposal, but make sure that you also listen to your body carefully. Don't ignore definite warning signs – the final chapter of this book will explain what to look out for – and if things don't quite go to plan always remind yourself that there will be another day.

Extreme fitness challenges are some of the most rewarding experiences there are, but nothing is worth sacrificing your long-term health. Furthermore, if your expectations are unrealistic and you don't meet them, you are more likely to become dispirited and give up. Play the long game, and let your achievements come naturally.

Overleaf: Whatever your personal challenge, fight to win.

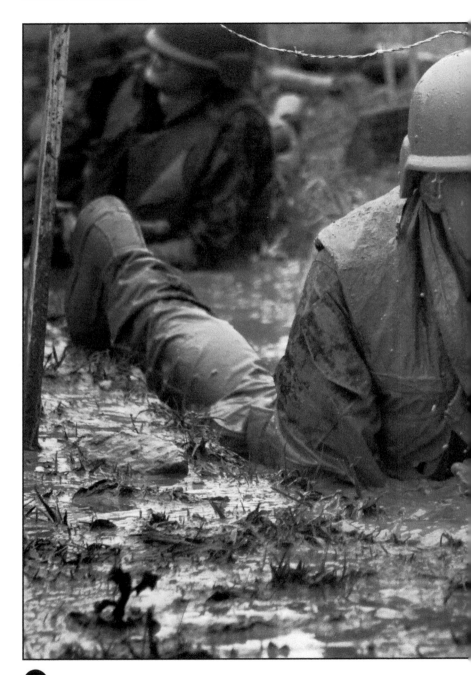

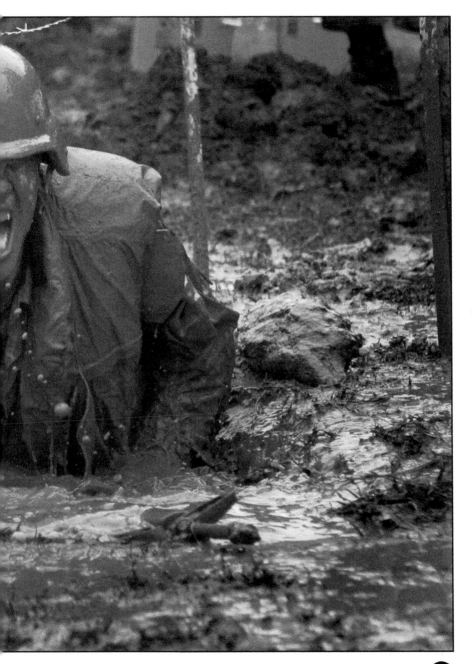

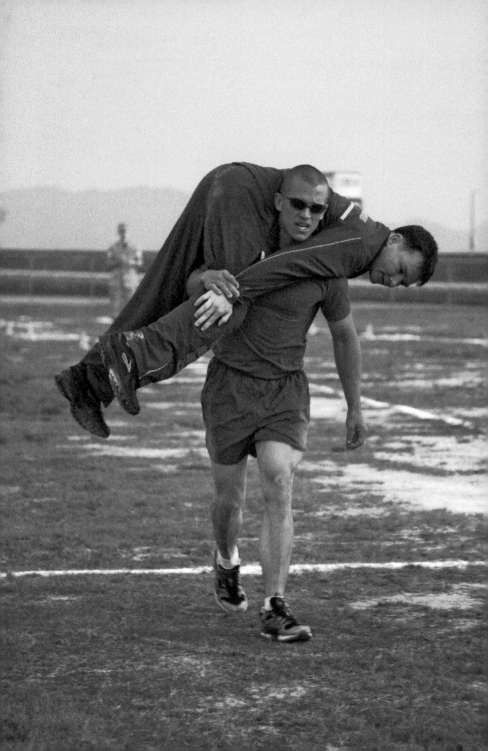

In the military world, non-combat injuries are one of the greatest threats to unit readiness at any one time. Military training and operations are hard on the body, placing huge demands on joints, muscles, tendons and ligaments, heart and lungs, and various other musculoskeletal components. On occasions, the body is unequal to the challenge and the result is an injury.

The numbers of people succumbing to injury, even in basic military training, are significant. One study, published in 2001, looked at injury rates among 756 men and 474 women in U.S. Army Basic Combat Training (BCT) at Fort Jackson, South Carolina. The total number of discharges (temporary or permanent) for injuries were 102 men and 108 women. As a general rule, around one in six recruits to any form of basic training will suffer an injury. However, in Special Forces training the rates of injury is far more worrisome. Classes of 100 candidates will typically lose 30 people to injury. Little wonder that the world of military health research is replete with papers on injury prevention and treatment.

The same health and injury problems afflict the world of civilian

8

Injuries are the curse of the endurance athlete. A sudden or progressive injury can bring a training programme or race to an abrupt halt, possibly indefinitely. As always, prevention is better than cure.

Injuries

. . . .
Opposite: Rehabilitating from an injury often takes a patient attitude and and clear recovery plan.

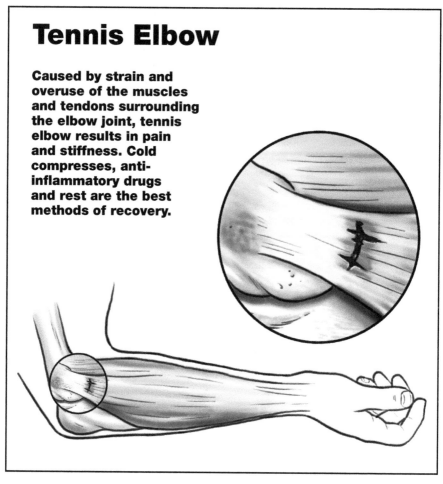

Tennis Elbow

Caused by strain and overuse of the muscles and tendons surrounding the elbow joint, tennis elbow results in pain and stiffness. Cold compresses, anti-inflammatory drugs and rest are the best methods of recovery.

sports, particularly those who train for and take part in major endurance feats. These problems can start young. In the United States, high-school athletes produce two million injuries and 500,000 doctor visits every year. Among adult athletes, nearly 70 per cent of runners will experience an injury at some point, and the rates are similarly high among other forms of sport.

Some injuries are obviously more serious than others. Blisters will heal naturally in a few days (unless they become infected for some reason), but a severely sprained ankle can stop training dead, possibly for many weeks. An injured knee or back could, more seriously, become a permanent bar to someone participating in a particular sport.

Injury Prevention

This chapter is not a detailed medical guide to preventing and treating sports injuries. Medical issues are complicated and require the hands-on treatment of a medical professional. Guide books such as these, and many others, are useful tools for suggesting a diagnosis, but should never act as a substitute for a proper consultation with a doctor or medical specialist. Rather, this chapter will focus mainly on the practicalities of injury prevention, plus look at the general principles of treating non-serious injuries, advice which should be taken in tandem with that of a qualified professional.

Taking Care

Like it or not, your body has limits. It is a physical object, and like any physical object it is subject to wear and tear, and the creeping attrition of age. So while this book recognizes that the body can be honed into a system capable of incredible athleticism, we also have to work within its natural restrictions if we are to avoid serious problems.

Here we issue a warning against overtraining. Pushing too hard for too long is all too easy for athletes with an intense desire to excel, but

at regular points the body needs to stop. This downtime is not a luxury. During rest periods, the body performs crucial repair functions, allowing it to strengthen and actually accrue the benefits of previous training sessions. The rest also provides a mental break, making you sharper and more focused when you return to the programme. If you overtrain, and never allow adequate rest, the problems will stack up. The *U.S. Navy SEAL Fitness Guide* lists some of the main characteristics of overtraining:

* *Decreased performance and muscle strength*
* *Decreased capacity to make decisions*
* *Burn-out or staleness*
* *Difficulty with concentration*
* *Chronically fatigued*
* *Angry and irritable*
* *Lacking motivation*
* *Muscle soreness*
* *Disturbances in mood*
* *Increased distractibility*
* *Feelings of depression*
* *Difficulty sleeping*
* *Change in heart rate at rest, exercise and recovery*
* *Increased susceptibility to colds or other illnesses*

– U.S. Navy, *U.S. Navy SEAL Fitness Guide*, p.216

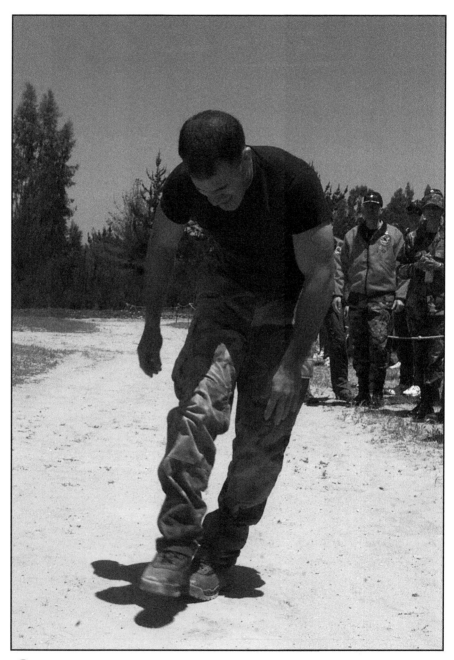

Opposite: Exhaustion can hit quickly, especially when combined with dehydration. Never keep training through chronic fatigue.

The guide's authors do note that there is no single laboratory test that can diagnose overtraining. The two most important indicators, however, are resting heart rate and mood.

In the exhausted athlete, resting heart rate in the morning (just after getting out of bed) is generally about 10–15bpm higher than his or her baseline resting rate. Combined with personality changes, the heart rate

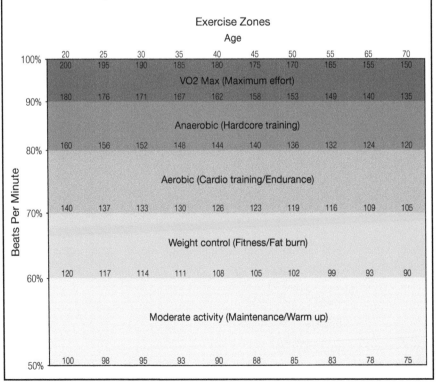

Heart Rate

The average resting heart rate of a man in his thirties is 71–75 beats per minute. For athletes, this can drop down to the 50s or even lower.

Exercise Zones

Age

	20	25	30	35	40	45	50	55	65	70
100%	200	195	190	185	180	175	170	165	155	150
				VO2 Max (Maximum effort)						
90%	180	176	171	167	162	158	153	149	140	135
				Anaerobic (Hardcore training)						
80%	160	156	152	148	144	140	136	132	124	120
				Aerobic (Cardio training/Endurance)						
70%	140	137	133	130	126	123	119	116	109	105
				Weight control (Fitness/Fat burn)						
60%	120	117	114	111	108	105	102	99	93	90
				Moderate activity (Maintenance/Warm up)						
50%	100	98	95	93	90	88	85	83	78	75

Beats Per Minute

Heart Rate Monitor

Monitors are useful for measuring heart rate at different stages of activity. Maximum heart rate should not be sustained for long during exercise.

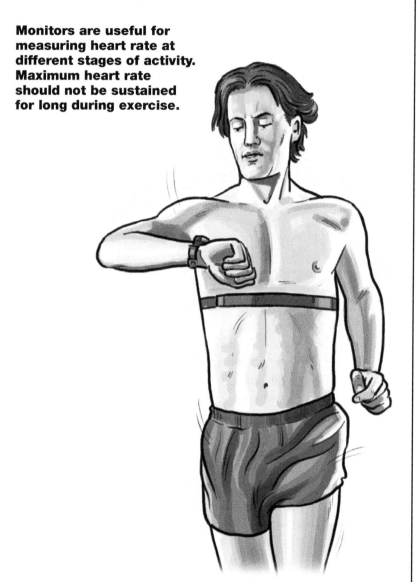

is a good indicator that the athlete's body desperately needs to recover. When training, you should also monitor your heart rate. Everyone has a maximum heart rate, and reaching and sustaining this rate is not advised for more than short periods. Everyone's max heart rate differs according to age and fitness, but the classic formula for calculating it is 220 minus age. This formula is not entirely accurate, and a good sports health check will provide you with a more accurate figure. As a general, and very important, point, if while running you start to feel sick, dizzy or have chest pains, stop immediately, rest and recover.

Dangers of Overtraining

Overtraining also dramatically increases your chances of suffering an injury. With the muscles weakened, and your attention levels suppressed, the possibilities of a twisted ankle, fall or worse are significantly higher. Fortunately, the prevention and treatment of overtraining is simple. First, ensure that you have adequate rest days in which you do no exercise whatsoever. You should have at least one rest day per week, with one or two light days of training between the high-intensity days. If no major race is in the offing, a policy of one day on, one day off is good for keeping injury

levels to a minimum. Eat properly on your rest days, and get fully hydrated. If muscles are sore, treat yourself with a professional sports massage, a warm bath or legs-up rest on a comfy sofa. Your goal is to get yourself to a refreshed state, fully energized to return to your training programme.

Another way to deal with overtraining is to practice cross-training. Switching to a different form of exercise means using different muscles in different ways, thereby breaking the repetitive actions of your regular sport. Cross-training, as Chapter 6 indicated, also gives your training regime a bit more colour and mental stimulus, keeping you psychologically fresh and less likely to lose interest in your training.

One point must be made with vigour. If you regularly experience pain, stiffness or heat in any part of your body, particularly the joints, don't ignore it and just keep training through it without consulting a doctor or specialist. I personally know several sportsmen who ignored the warning signs and pushed through injuries that steadily increased in their severity. The ultimate outcome was avoidable surgery and an end to their pursuit of that particular sport. The moral is – look after your body, and don't be a hero if you suspect you have an injury.

Running Injuries

Running can induce a range of physical problems, highlighted here. Correct running posture, good footwear and recovery time are the keys to prevention.

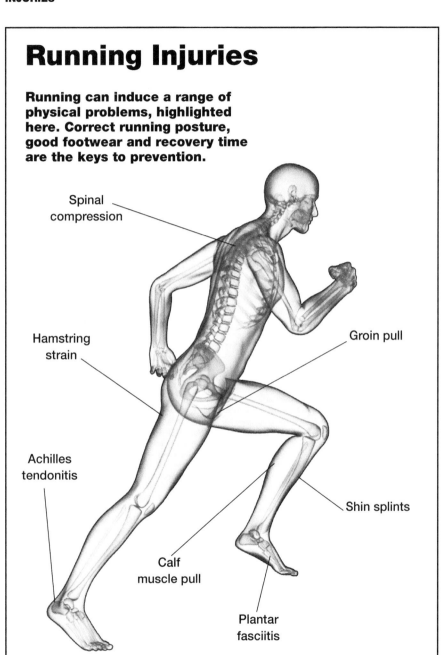

Spinal compression

Hamstring strain

Groin pull

Achilles tendonitis

Shin splints

Calf muscle pull

Plantar fasciitis

Common Injuries

The phrase 'common injuries' contains a broad spectrum of complaints, from the relatively trivial to significant joint injuries. Note that certain sports, and certain techniques within certain sports, have their own set of injuries associated with them. In weight training, for example, the five most common injuries are:

- Muscle strain
- Shoulder impingement (the result of inflamed shoulder muscles)
- Disc herniation
- Ligament sprain
- Muscle contusion

As we would expect, this list of injuries are principally the result of stress-loading, occurring when muscles, ligaments and various other physical components are put under heavy pressure. In running sports, we would naturally expect many of the most common injuries to be of the repetitive strain variety, concentrated in the lower limbs. Here the *U.S. Navy SEAL Fitness Guide* provides a list of these injuries, based on those experienced during training programmes and operations:

The list in the left column is the stuff of nightmares for committed runners, and at one point in a running career all runners will typically suffer

Plantar fasciitis	Inflammation and tightness of thick fibrous band on sole of foot.
Achilles tendonitis	Inflammation of calf tendon or 'heel cords' especially at insertion into heel.
Iliotibial band rub	Pain on outside or lateral aspect of knee or high on outside of the hip.
Bursitis	Inflammation or irritation of various bursal sacs about inner or medial portion of knee, or behind the heel.
Shin splints	Pain along medial aspect of lower third of tibia, worse in morning, resolves after warming up. Resolves with cooling down after running.
Back strain/sprain	Results from impact loading of spine.

– U.S. Navy, *U.S. Navy SEAL Fitness Guide*, p.214

Injuries to the Feet

The foot is a complex network of muscles, tendons and bones. Foot injuries range from blisters to serious sprains or breaks. Warm the foot up with gentle rotary motions before exercise.

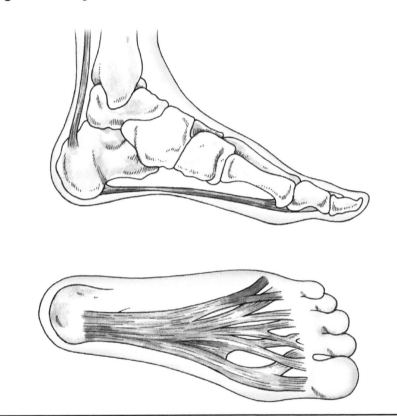

from one or more of them. Runners, like all sportsmen, should become familiar not only with the injuries endemic to their sport, but also the prevention strategies available. There are many excellent sports-injury prevention manuals on the market, and doing some research into the issues could make the difference between safe and dangerous training.

Blisters

Before looking at some of the more serious categories of sporting injury, we start small with an injury that bedevils almost all endurance athletes at times – the blister. Blisters are essentially the result of friction burns. When a patch of skin suffers repeated friction, it responds by producing fluid. This fluid builds up under the skin, causing the distinctive dome-shaped blister. Blisters are non-serious, but they can be excruciatingly painful and race-wrecking in their larger and more developed forms. They can also, if allowed to burst and get dirty, become infected and require more substantial medical treatment, so they need to be treated with care.

Blisters are most common on the feet in running sports, the feet experiencing hours of friction inside socks and sports shoes, but they can also affect the hands in sports such as cycling or rock climbing, or other parts of the body where there is friction contact between clothing and skin. Here are some key tips for preventing foot blisters in particular:

• Moisturize your feet – the drier the foot, the more susceptible it is to friction and blisters. You should apply moisturizer on a daily basis, then a special skin lubricant on race days.

Vaseline will do, but you can also buy specific running products.
• Make sure your shoes and socks fit perfectly. Neither should be too tight, nor should the socks have an excess fabric building up around the toes or heel. You can also try wearing two pairs of thin socks; the double layer reduces the friction between the foot and the shoe.
• Tape up – for some endurance races, apply self-adhesive medical tape to the potential problem areas.

If you do get a blister, and it is small and unobtrusive, then simply allowing it to heal may be the best course of action. For larger blisters interfering with your movements, bursting is the best option. Take a needle and sterilize it with alcohol. (Don't sterilize it with an open flame, as the needle will pick up carbon particles that it will then transfer into the blister.) Take the needle and insert a small hole at a point around the blister's base, so that fluid starts to ooze out. Now apply direct pressure to the body of the blister with a sterile pad to force out all the fluid. Once this is complete, cover the blister with a bandage.

Sprains and Strains

Here we are going to use 'sprains and strains' to cover any sudden-

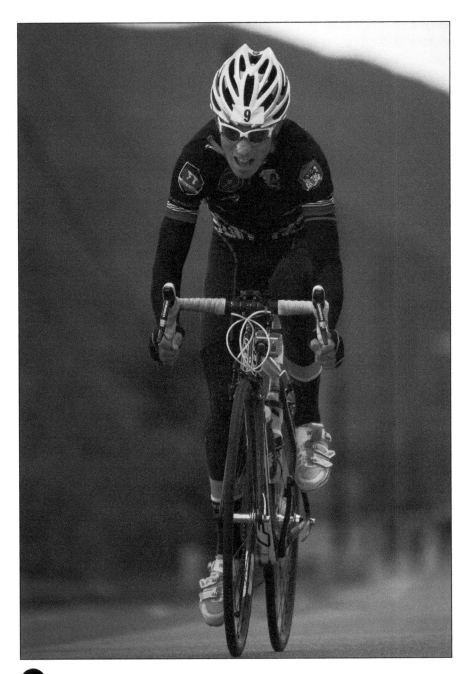

Opposite: When cycling, always wear a high-quality helmet offering full skull protection.

onset musculoskeletal injury, such as a twisted ankle or knee. In terms of the very basic treatments described below, you should recognize that these are immediate actions only, and that proper medical help is required.

Preventing sprains and strains requires a range of measures, both mental and physical. First, try to avoid conducting intense exercise while you are very tired. Fatigue weakens muscle control, and also leads to the inattention that can cause slips and falls when running. If your training takes you over uneven surfaces – such as those typically encountered during hill running – look well ahead and identify potential hazards in advance. Choose your footing carefully and slow down to a comfortable level when negotiating difficult sections of a course.

A proper warm-up will also help with sprain prevention, as will investing in good equipment, particularly running shoes. Make sure

U.S. Navy SEALs Tip – Treating Muscle Cramps

Muscle cramps are common and may be precipitated by prolonged physical activity, high heat and humidity (black flag conditions), dehydration and/or poor conditioning. Cramps are characterized by the sudden onset of moderately severe to incapacitating pain in the muscle belly and may progress to involve other adjacent muscle groups. The first treatment consists of immediate rehydration with a fluid containing electrolytes. After beginning rehydration, further treatment should consist of grasping and applying pressure to the muscle belly and immediately putting the muscle on stretch until the cramp resolves. The calf muscle, for example, would be stretched by flexing the foot toward the head, whereas a thigh cramp would be treated by flexing the knee, bringing the foot to the buttocks.

– U.S. Navy, *U.S. Navy SEAL Fitness Guide*, p.208

Sprained Ankle

A common injury from running on uneven surfaces, an ankle sprain occurs when a ligament has been twisted or stretched beyond its natural limits.

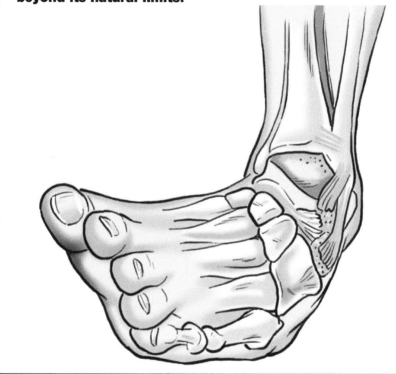

that these are properly fitted and laced up, and that you have tested them on forgiving surfaces before you venture on to anything more challenging. If you have suffered sprains before, the likelihood is that the affected joint is permanently weakened and will therefore be vulnerable to future injury. With the help of a qualified physiotherapist, use progressive and targeted weight training and range-of-motion (ROM) exercises to restore the joint to strength. If you are in the recovery phase of an injury, introduce the limb back to exercise gently, and stop if

Tearing a Ligament

Torn knee ligaments can lead to cartilage damage and even osteoarthritis if not given sufficient time to heal.

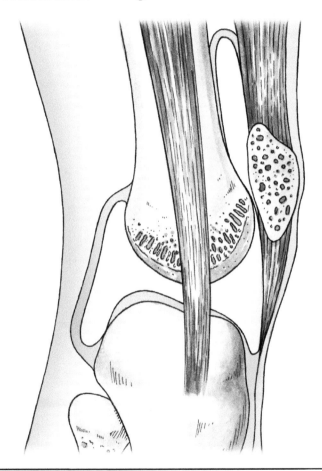

you start to experience significant pain or a sense of weakness returning. In fact, as a general point don't ignore any sort of pain build up. My attempts once to run through an aching lower back resulted in a properly pulled back miles from home, and a humiliating hobble

Physiotherapy

Physical therapy can both ease and avert injuries. Make sure your physiotherapist is properly accredited and trained specifically in treating sports injuries.

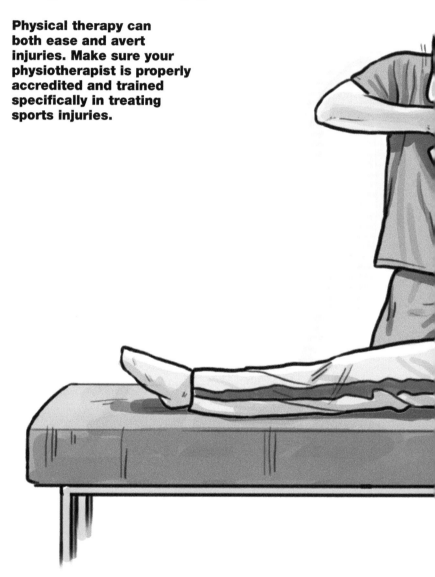

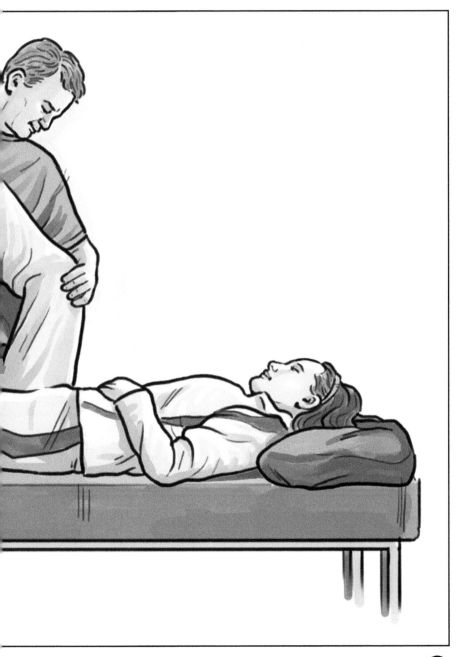

Compression Sleeves

Compression support can prevent further damage to injuries as well as helping recovery. However, a health professional should always be consulted if pain does not ease.

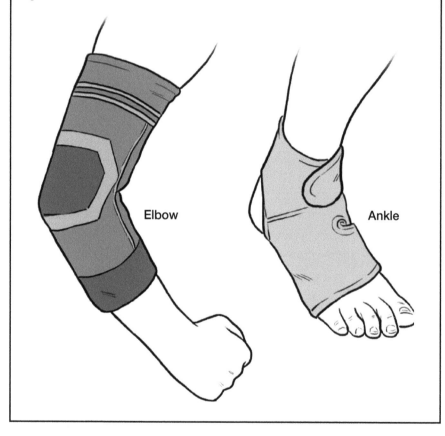

Elbow

Ankle

back. You can also protect vulnerable joints by wearing an appropriate compression support, or by taping up the joint with elastic bandage. Make sure that neither the support nor the bandage restrict the joint's full movement.

Certainly the most significant measure you can implement to prevent debilitating sprains and

U.S. Navy SEALs Advice – Common Swimming Injuries

Freestyle, butterfly and backstroke place a great amount of stress on the shoulder joint. Use alternate or bilateral breathing on freestyle and be sure to get plenty of roll on backstroke. Before beginning a butterfly set, be sure you are well warmed up. This will allow the shoulder to stay in a more neutral position during the activity of arm recovery and this neutral position helps prevent what is known as 'impingement syndrome'.

Freestyle swimming and kicking with a kickboard places a great amount of stress on the low back because of hyperextension; doing the backstroke relieves the stress. A pullbuoy is also helpful as it raises the hips and allows the spine to assume a more neutral posture.

Kicking with fins may aggravate the knee (especially the knee cap) and result in a degenerative condition known as patellofemoral syndrome, which commonly afflicts athletic individuals.

The breaststroke kick helps balance the knee joint by increasing muscular tone on the inside of the quadriceps muscle, and serves to balance the effect that running has: increasing muscular tone on the outside portion of the quadriceps muscle. However, the breaststroke may actually intensify iliotibial band syndrome. Swimmers may need to avoid doing breaststroke if they feel increased pain over the outside of the knee.

strains is to have good technique in whatever you do. Ensure that you have correct posture, particularly in terms of head–neck–spine alignment, and observe closely if you have any areas of tension developing.

Any injury to musculoskeletal tissue results in an instant body reaction to protect the injured site. One of the main mechanisms is inflammation, the injured site swelling up (signified by redness, bruising and tissue expansion). Although the swelling mechanism is by its nature protective, problems arise if it is allowed to continue beyond

RICE Procedure

The RICE procedure is excellent for treating minor injuries that result in swelling. Avoid putting excess weight on the swollen limb during the healing process.

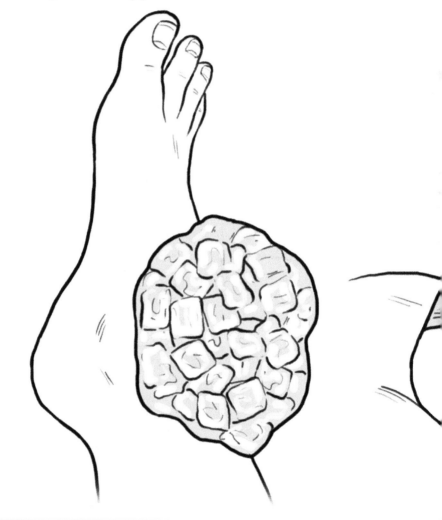

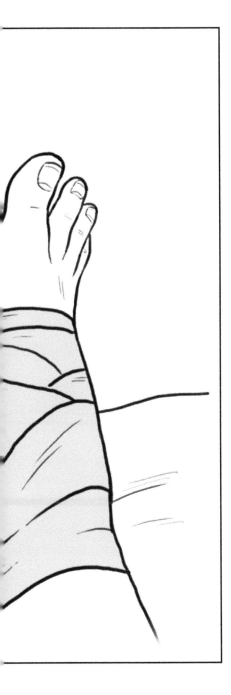

acceptable limits. Uncontrolled swelling leads to the tissue becoming congested and extremely painful, and the inflammation also restricts an injured joint's full ROM.

In terms of basic first aid, the priority for treating such injuries is to control the inflammatory reaction through external means. (Important note: what appears to be a sprained joint could actually be a fracture. For any severe sprain injury, you should attend a hospital immediately and have the joint x-rayed to assess the damage fully.) The tried and tested method for treating injuries of this nature is remembered by the mnemonic 'RICE':

- **R**est
- **I**ce
- **C**ompression
- **E**levation

The components of this response break down as follows, according to the U.S. Navy SEALs:

'REST' *means applying no weight or only partial weight to the extremity; crutches should be used for locomotion. 'Relative rest' means decreasing activities that cause pain and replacing them with other activities that are pain-free.*

'ICE' means applying ice. This should continue until swelling has stabilized. [Important: Don't apply ice for more than 20 minutes to an injured joint area, as you run the risk of inducing frostbite.]

'COMPRESSION' means applying an Ace wrap or similar compression wrap to the injured part for periods of 2–4 hours. Never sleep with a compression wrap applied unless medically advised.

'ELEVATION' means placing the injured part above the level of the heart; this allows gravity to help reduce swelling and fluid accumulation.

– U.S. Navy, *U.S. Navy SEAL Fitness Guide*, p.200–01

The RICE procedure has the ultimate goal of reducing the swelling to manageable levels, and giving the injured body part as little movement as possible. The subsequent rehabilitation of the injured joint (under professional medical guidance) then typically focuses on gently returning the full ROM through controlled exercises. Injured-ankle ROM exercises include:

The alphabet – with the foot dangling free, slowly draw all the letters of the alphabet in the air with your big toe, keeping the shin static. Make the letters as large as your joint will allow.

Foot turns and points – moving only your ankle, put your foot into a range of positions: pointing upward; pointing downward; turned inward; turned outward. Hold each position for 15 seconds before returning to the neutral position.

Towel pull – hook a towel around the front of your foot and pull it gently upwards to draw back the foot. Again, keep the leg static as you do this exercise and hold the pull for 15 seconds before returning to the neutral position.

You can assist injury recover with anti-inflammatory medications, of course. Some of these, such as ibuprofen or asprin, are readily available over the counter in pharmacies and supermarkets, while more powerful varieties will require a prescription from a doctor. Some anti-inflammatories can exacerbate other medical conditions, such as high blood pressure, so take medical advice before beginning any course of medication.

The RICE and ROM techniques will return many sprained joints to full function. Signs that all is well include the joint having full ROM with no pain, can take weight comfortably and experiences no symptoms of weakness. However, if problems persist over a long period, it may be a sign that more interventionist medical treatments are required, including surgery.

Heat Stroke

As this book has frequently discussed, extreme fitness challenges can take people into remote and sometimes dangerous terrains, exposing them to adverse climates. Space does not allow us to consider the full spectrum of medical emergencies, but one requires special consideration – hyperthermia. The loss of no fewer than three SAS candidates during summer 2013 selection training reminds us that even superbly fit young individuals can succumb to this potentially lethal condition, and anyone involved in extreme sports needs to be able to spot the warning signs in themselves and others.

Hypothermia – a life-threatening drop in the core body temperature – has already been introduced in Chapter 4 in the context of aquatic sports. Out of water, the most dangerous threat to many

U.S. Navy SEAL Tip – Applying Ice

All soft tissue or joint injuries, except open wounds, will benefit by immediate application of ice. It can be applied either passively or actively. Passive application is when you take some form of ice: crushed ice, ice slush, an ice pack or snow and apply it to the injured body part. Active application is when you take the ice (perhaps in water frozen in a cup or bag) and massage the injured part with it. At home, a bag of frozen peas is an excellent way to passively ice the injured part, as the peas easily conform to the swollen area. After 20 minutes, the bag of peas can be tossed back into the freezer for reapplication later. The normal response to ice includes cold, burning, aching and finally numbness over the affected part. This progression occurs over 7–10 minutes

– U.S. Navy, *U.S. Navy SEAL Fitness Guide*, p.201

Treating Heatstroke

Cooling the body is paramount when treating heatstroke. Keep the patient calm (heastroke can produce confusion or aggression) and soak the clothing and skin with cool water.

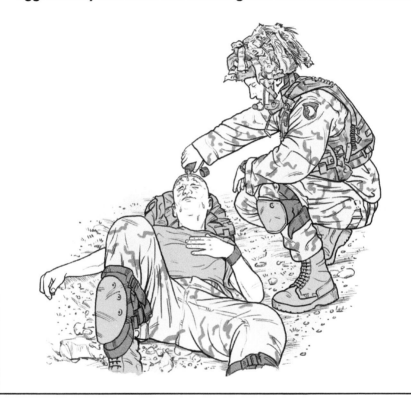

adventurous sportsmen and women is hyperthermia, when the body essentially produces more heat than it actually dissipates, which is a potentially life-threatening condition. Runners and other endurance sports enthusiasts are particularly exposed to this threat, especially if they raise their body temperature through intense exercise while also being exposed to strong external heat from the sun. Combine this effect with dehydration and the mixture is potentially lethal.

Spotting Hyperthermia

Signs of hyperthermia include excessive sweating, dilated pupils and hot, dry skin. Try to prevent the patient losing conciousness at all costs.

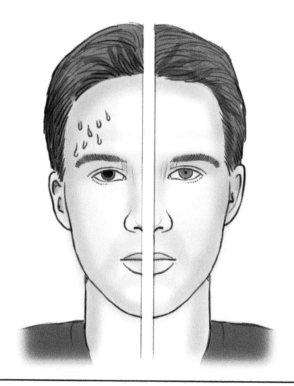

Hyperthermia has two phases – heat exhaustion and heat stroke. Heat exhaustion occurs when the core body temperature climbs between 37°C (98.6°F) and 40°C (104°F), resulting in the body's levels of water and salt beginning to drop.

The symptoms of this mounting problem are dizziness, nausea, profuse sweating and confusion. As soon as they occur, you should get yourself (or the affected third party) into the shade quickly, take off any excess clothing, rehydrate thoroughly

Performing Triage

Triage is a system of ascertaining the severity of injuries and the order in which patients are treated. If several people are in need of treatment, triage is performed to decide who should receive immediate attention.

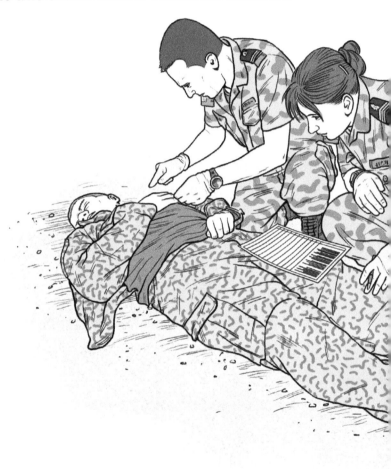

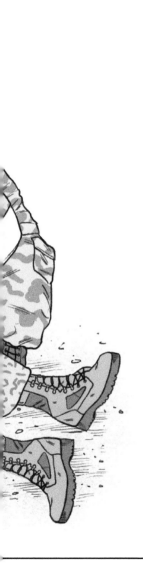

with frequent sips of fluid (drink water or sports drinks, and avoid alcohol or caffeine) and moisten the skin repeatedly with cool water (the process of evaporation from the skin assists with body cooling). All being well, you should respond to this treatment within 30 minutes. Anyone who doesn't, and whose condition actually worsens, is likely to be moving into a state of heat stroke.

With heat stroke, the body's core temperature now climbs above 40°C (104°F). The symptoms of heat stroke include:

• Very hot skin that feels 'flushed'
• Increasing dizziness and lapses of consciousness
• Heavy sweating that suddenly stops, resulting in dry skin
• Oppressive fatigue
• Muscle cramps
• Feeling or being sick
• A rapid heartbeat
• Mental confusion, including hallucinations and lack of coordination
• Seizures
• Urinating infrequently, and exhibiting dark urine.

If heat stroke is left untreated, the casualty will suffer organ failure, coma and eventually death. It is a medical emergency requiring immediate hospitalization. Before help arrives, treatment is largely that described for heat exhaustion, but more intensively

Checking a Pulse

Check a pulse at the radial artery in the wrist or the carotid artery of the neck, on each side of the windpipe. Use the first two fingers as pictured, avoiding the thumb as it has its own pulse.

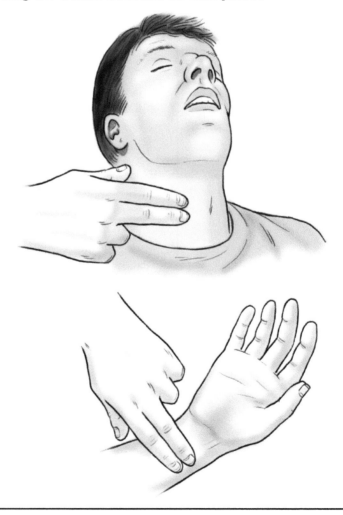

applied. Soak the skin constantly with cool (not cold) water, and fan the skin to encourage more rapid evaporation. (Israeli Special Forces sometimes carry water mist sprays, this being a good way to distribute the water evenly over the skin.) You can also massage the skin very gently to stimulate the now-sluggish circulation. Don't give medications, even common ones such as paracetamol and asprin, and place the casualty in the recovery position.

Heat exhaustion and heat stroke are very serious conditions, and during any endurance race (especially one in a hot climate) you should keep a close eye on others as well as yourself. The important point is to stop heat exhaustion in its tracks as soon as it begins to develop. Don't let it get too far advanced, as then it may well have gone too far to stop.

Anyone who participates in extreme sports will likely suffer injuries from time to time. With care and adequate time for recovery, most of these injuries will pass and not prevent the individual from going on to have a long sporting career.

U.S. Army Tips – Hydration

- Drink cool (4.4°C/40°F) water. This is the best drink to sustain performance. Fluid also comes from juice, milk, soup and other beverages.
- Do not drink coffee, tea and soft drinks even though they provide fluids. The caffeine in them acts as a diuretic that can increase urine production and fluid loss. Avoid alcohol for the same reason.
- Drink large quantities of water one or two hours before exercise to promote hyperhydration. This allows time for adequate hydration and urination.
- Drink three to six ounces [85–170ml] of fluid every 15 to 30 minutes during exercise.
- Replace fluid sweat losses by monitoring pre- and post-exercise body weights. Drink two cups of fluid for every pound of weight lost.

– FM 21-20, *Physical Fitness Guide*, 6-5

Glossary

Adductor: muscle that pulls a body part towards the body, such as in the thigh, arm, toe or finger (opposite to abductor muscle, which draws the body part away from the body)

Adrenaline: also known as epinephrine, adrenaline is a hormone produced during exercise that flows through the nervous system and prepares the muscles for action

Aerobic: literally meaning the use or presence of oxygen, aerobic exercise is that for which the body can supply enough oxygen, such as running or swimming

Anaerobic: high-intensity exercise that uses up more oxygen than the body can take in (hence it literally means 'without oxygen'), triggering the release of lactic acid, which ferments and turns glucose into energy. This occurs during exercises such as weight lifting and calisthenics.

Bar bell: weighted discs on the end of a long handle, which can be detached or added for resistance training

Bench press: lifting weights from a prone position, lying on the back and pushing the weight upwards until the arms are straight, before lowering the weight to the chest

Blood pressure: measurement of how hard your heart has to work to pump blood through vessels; the lower the blood pressure, the lower your heart has to work

BMI (body mass index): the percentages of fat, muscle, skeleton and organs that make up a person's total weight

Calisthenics: exercises designed to promote flexibility and strength, generally performed without weights, such as sit-ups, press-ups or lunges

Calorie: measurement of food energy in a food or drink product

Circuit training: undertaking a variety of exercises on one exercise apparatus or station, followed by a series of exercises to develop strength and stamina

Crunch: also known as sit-ups, crunches work the abdominal muscles by curling the upper body upwards to meet the knees

Dead lift: lifting a weight off the floor to waist height, bending the knees and keeping the back straight

Electrolytes: essential salts, including sodium and potassium, necessary to avoid dehydration

Hyperthermia: a state when the core of the body becomes too hot due to its inability to dispel more heat than it absorbs; it is often a side effect of extreme exertion in hot conditions

Ligament: tissues connecting bones or cartilage to surrounding muscles

Lunge: stretching the quad, hamstring and glute muscles by pushing the weight forward onto one foot and bending the corresponding knee

Maximum heart rate: highest number of beats per minute (BPM) the heart rate safely reaches during physical exercise

Meditation: also known as mindfulness, meditation is a way of relaxing the mind to promote wellbeing and avoid stress-related health problems

Metabolic rate: rate in which the body burns food energy, which is stored as fat if it is not burned off with exercise

Power rack: also known as a power cage, the rack allows single person use of weights, with bar catchers built in for safety

Press-up: also known as push-ups, press-ups use the arms to lower and raise the body, working the abdominals and arm muscles

Resistance training: building muscle strength and size by weight lifting, increasing the weight and force on the muscle over time

Squat: from a standing position, bend the knees to lower the torso towards the ground, keeping the back straight, before returning to standing position this reduces barrel distortion and improves accuracy.

INDEX

Page numbers in *italics* refer to illustrations.